Chil[illegible] Cancer
Understanding and Coping

Childhood Cancer

Understanding and Coping

HENRY EKERT

Director
Department of Haematology and Oncology
Royal Children's Hospital
Melbourne, Australia

GORDON AND BREACH SCIENCE PUBLISHERS
New York • Philadelphia • London • Paris • Montreux • Tokyo • Melbourne

Published 1989
Second Printing 1990

Gordon and Breach Science Publishers

Post Office Box 786
Cooper Station
New York, New York 10276
United States of America

5301 Tacony Street, Slot 330
Philadelphia, Pennsylvania 19137
United States of America

Post Office Box 197
London WC2E 9PX
England

58, rue Lhomond
75005 Paris
France

Post Office Box 161
1820 Montreux 2
Switzerland

3-14-9, Okubo
Shinjuku-ku, Tokyo 169
Japan

Private Bag 8
Camberwell, Victoria 3124
Australia

Library of Congress Cataloging-in-Publication Data

Ekert, Henry.
Childhood cancer.

Bibliography: p.
Includes index.
1. Tumors in children—Psychological aspects.
2. Adjustment (Psychology) I. Title.
RC281.C4E34 1989 618.92′994 89-11691
ISBN ~~2-88124-356-8~~

Chapter 9: The Dying Child 63

SPECIFIC CONDITIONS

Chapter 10: Acute Lymphocytic Leukemia—ALL 73

Preface

This book has been written to provide information for parents, relatives and friends of children and adolescents with cancer. It is also suitable for health professionals who work with such children and adolescents.

The book gives the reader an outline of the causes, incidence and types of childhood cancer. The concept of chance as the major cause of cancer is explained. The process by which the diagnosis is established and the extent of tumor determined is described in general and specific terms. The choice of treatment methods and their short and long term results are discussed. The role of modern technology, such as bone marrow transplantation and developments arising from genetic engineering, which are relevant to childhood cancer, are also described.

The reader is given an understanding of the complex emotional responses which invariably accompany the diagnosis of cancer in children. The stress accompanying treatment is discussed, as well as the emotional needs and responses at times of crisis, such as recurrence or death. Support for the dying child and measures which can be used to reduce pain and anxiety are described. Guidelines are offered on how to explain to children, cancer and the methods used for its treatment.

No attempt has been made to recommend or describe details of specific types of treatment. Rather, the general principles of treatment with chemotherapy, surgery and irradiation are outlined for each tumor and their advantages and disadvantages discussed. In this way, the book should complement and reinforce medical advice given at treatment centers and act as a reference to remind the family of some of the facts and details about their child's illness. It may also prove useful in helping them make difficult decisions when a crisis arises during treatment or at relapse.

The scientific and medical facts about childhood cancer are integrated with the emotional impact of the disease on the child and the family. There is an overall message of hope and optimism without minimizing the serious nature of the disease and its treatment.

Acknowledgements

First, foremost, I wish to thank the patients and families of children with cancer whose feelings and comments as expressed to me in interviews over many years have inspired me to write this book. I also wish to thank my medical, nursing, and allied health professional colleagues for their helpful comments and discussion.

My special thanks go to Dr. R. Y. Mathew who gave most generously of his time to review the manuscript. He has constantly urged me to express clearly the scientific and medical concepts described in this book and to be brief. If I have failed to do so it is no fault of his.

I would also like to thank Mrs. Jan Murphy and Dr. Thomas Fok, without whose valuable secretarial assistance this book with its illustrations could not have been produced. Last, but not least, I wish to thank my family who supported me in this enterprise.

General Topics

CHAPTER 1

Causes of Childhood Cancer

CHILDHOOD CANCER: THE CONCEPT OF CHANCE

Most people accept that in the middle or late stages of life the body may malfunction, resulting in a variety of diseases. Cancer at this stage of life is often viewed as the response of the body to abuses of the environment or life styles. The relationship between cigarette smoking and lung cancer, or certain types of diet and bowel cancer, are the best known examples of environmental cancers. It is this type of reasoning that leads one to look at the child's environment and the family's life style and to try to find something that may have caused the cancer. In childhood cancer this type of logic does not apply because, with few exceptions, there has been insufficient time for environmental factors to cause cancer.

The great majority of children's cancers should be considered as a special form of congenital malformations comparable to the cleft lip and palate or spina-bifida.

Each person begins as the joining of two cells, the ovum and the sperm into one cell which then contains the full complement of inherited material derived from the mother's ovum and the father's sperm. This single cell commences to divide and continues to do so until eventually after billions of divisions there are sufficient numbers of cells to form the rudiments of all the complicated organs of the body. Division of the cells requires that the inheritance chemical material known as DNA (deoxyribose nucleic acid) be organized into structures known as the chromosomes, that these be doubled and then equally distributed to the daughter cells. Each DNA molecule consists of a 5 carbon sugar called deoxyribose to which are attached a phosphate molecule and a nitrogenous base. The nitrogenous bases are one of 4 types, adenine, guanine, cytosine and thymine. The DNA molecules are arranged in long chains along the chromosome. This long chain arrangement is formed by chemical links between the phosphate of one DNA molecule to the sugar of the next molecule upstream from it. This arrangement is shown below:

```
phosphate — Sugar — phosphate — Sugar — phosphate
              |                   |
             base                base
```

The DNA on the chromosomes exists as 2 chains twisted around each other in the form a double stranded helix. The 2 chains are linked to each other by chemical bonds between the bases. These chemical bonds only form between adenine and thymine and between guanine and cytosine. The sequence of the bases on the DNA chain of the chromosome are the genetic code of the individual which determine the structure and function of all cells. The structure of DNA is shown in Figure 1. Prior to cell division, the quantity of DNA in the nucleus doubles and the chromosomes containing the DNA split into two chains which are arranged in the center of the cell along a tubular system of proteins called the spindle. The cell then divides into 2 daughter cells each containing one complete set of chromosomes with its DNA. This process is diagramatically illustrated in Figure 2.

The duplication of DNA and its distribution to the daughter cells requires generation of energy and involves a variety of complicated chemical reactions regulated by enzymes. *Purely by chance* it is certain that some errors in this process will occur. Some of the cells in which such an error has taken place may die but others may survive and remain dormant.

Specialization of Function—"Differentiation"

In addition to multiplication of cells to form the various organs of the body the cells also develop specialist functions. They are programmed to become skin, muscle, bone and brain. This is called differentiation, and is closely linked with multiplication. In general, multiplication stops when differentiation begins.

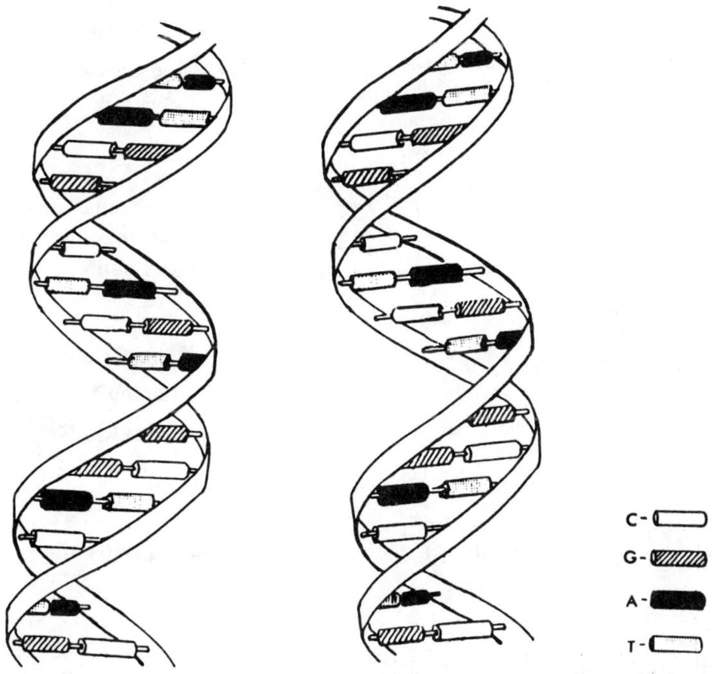

FIGURE 1 Double helix structure of DNA. The structure of DNA is shown as two chains held together by bonds between bases represented as T(thymine), A(adenine), G(guanine) and C(cytosine). The bonds are formed between T and A and G and C. The sequence of the bases on the double helix structure acts as a code which governs cell behaviour.

When differentiation is faulty, malformations of organs can occur giving rise to well known congenital malformations such as spina bifida.

Genetic Changes Leading to Cancer

Dormant cells with an error in their genetic material may by chance have an error which confers a growth advantage on the cells. As a result these cell will continue to multiply rather than differentiate. In the environment of a developing embryo however, there are powerful forces stimulating differentiation rather than multiplication. These forces are sufficiently power-

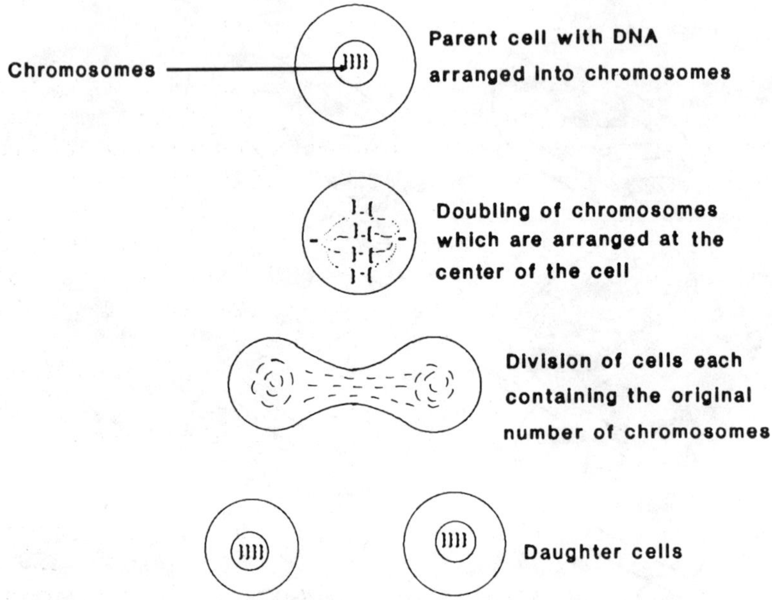

FIGURE 2 Stages of cell division.

ful to overcome the urge of the dormant cell to proliferate. These cells may remain in the organs of the body in much the same way as an underground mine, ready to explode if triggered by some other stimulus or simply through ageing. With increasing age after birth the body's drive towards differentiation of cells diminishes as all the organs have been formed. They will now simply grow in size, either by growth in size of cells or by an ordered multiplication followed by differentiation of selected primitive cells such as those of the bone marrow, immune system or gut.

It is easy to see how the dormant cells with their multiplication potential, when freed from the drive to differentiate, are ready to revert to multiplying cells. These cells are childhood cancer cells and their unrestricted growth gives rise to childhood cancer. Considering the billions of cell multiplications that give rise to the human body and the relative rarity of childhood cancer it is a marvel that childhood cancers are so rare.

Evidence for Genetic and Chance Causes of Cancer

Studies with highly specific antibodies directed to various stages of cell differentiation, together with advances in more detailed studies of chromosome appearances and gene arrangements have allowed a new understanding of the cause of childhood cancer. In leukemia, research using a variety of antibodies has shown that the leukemic cells have features characteristic of certain stages of early differentiation from primitive cells to mature normal bone marrow cells. In growing numbers of solid tumors such as Wilms', Retinoblastoma and Ewing's sarcoma there are specific genetic changes in the tumor cells which are not present in adjoining normal cells. These genetic changes can sometimes be associated with the production of growth factors which stimulate these cells to multiply rather than to differentiate. Changes in the genetic material can also be demonstrated in a very high proportion of leukemia cells, and these changes often go hand in hand with the rate of growth and structural features of these cells. In some cancers there is a loss of genetic material in a symmetrical fashion on both chromosomes, and this loss allows the cell to grow in an uncontrolled manner.

All these lines of evidence are still indirect, but for the first time they permit construction of a reasonable proposition, backed by established facts, of the relationship between cell behavior and its genetic material. With time, more and more blanks of the jigsaw puzzle will be filled in by further scientific research.

At this stage of our knowledge it is possible to view childhood cancer as a congenital malformation. With this understanding the question of "whose fault?" becomes irrelevant because chance is nobody's fault. The concept of genetic changes which can lead to cancer is illustrated in Figure 3.

ENVIRONMENTAL FACTORS

Concern is expressed in the press and by community groups and individuals about environmental factors which they claim can cause childhood cancer. It is necessary to distinguish between those claims that have been scientifically established as

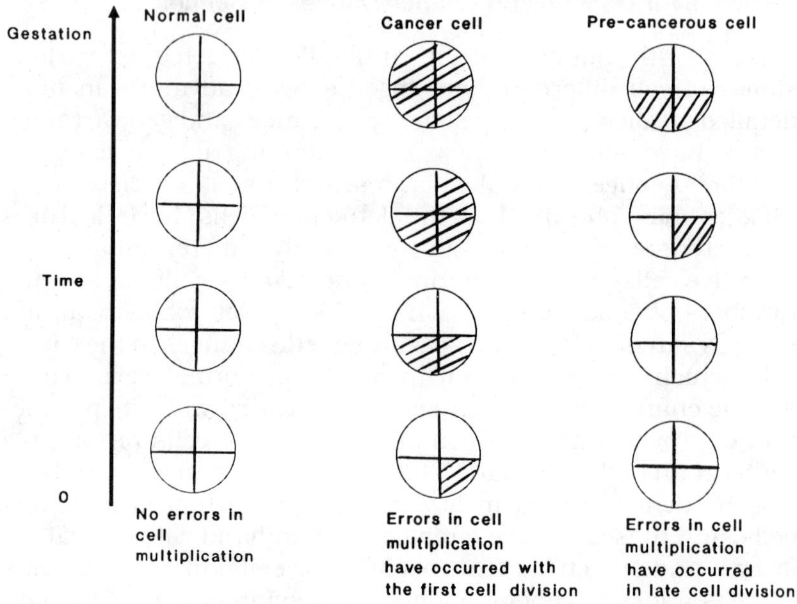

FIGURE 3 Possible mechanism of genetic changes (mutation) which can give rise to cancer.

a cause of cancer from those which may be used for political purposes by people with a particular point of view.

Radiation

There is no doubt that radiation can cause cancer if the person is exposed to it in a big enough dose or at a vulnerable time. Radiation exposure during the first 3 months of pregnancy is one of the established causes of childhood leukemia. Exposure to radiation may have occurred for medical reasons such as an x-ray of the abdomen in early pregnancy, or due to environmental irradiation e.g. from radiation as a result of a nuclear accident. It is not impossible that an increase in radioactivity in the proximity of a nuclear power station could also cause an increase in childhood cancer if this increase of radioactivity occurred during a critical stage of development of the embryo. Conclusive proof that this has actually happened is lacking.

While there is undeniable proof that x-rays in early pregnancy can cause childhood leukemia, there is absolutely no evidence that ultrasound examinations can cause cancers. So many of these have been performed that one can be certain that if there were any association between ultrasound examinations and childhood cancer this would by now have been observed.

Recently the safety of above ground high voltage power lines has been questioned. It is claimed that the electromagnetic fields produced by these high voltages can induce childhood leukemia. This concept has been put forward by certain community groups and evidence has been sought by epidemiologic studies. So far no evidence has been presented that the incidence of leukemia in the vicinity of high voltage power lines is greater than may have occurred by chance.

Chemicals

Insecticide and weedicide sprays have also been claimed by some to cause childhood cancer. The evidence is very sparse. Certainly these substances can cause damage to genetic material when they are present in high concentrations. It is conceivable that, as with radiation, if these chemicals are present in high concentration in early pregnancy they could damage genetic material. There is however, no proof that this is a significant cause of childhood cancer.

Drugs and Hormones

Hormones and drugs given in early pregnancy have been incriminated in congenital malformations. Could they also be a cause of cancer in children? One hormone which was once given in early pregnancy namely diethylstilbesterol has been definitely shown to be associated with an increased risk of developing a special form of vaginal cancer in young women. No other hormone or medically prescribed drug has been shown to be associated with an increased risk of cancer in childhood.

FAMILIAL TENDENCY TO CANCER

Some rare congenital conditions which are diagnosed in early childhood make the individual cancer prone. These are well recognized and long lists of them are available but they are very rare. Individual families with these conditions are warned by their doctors that they may be susceptible to cancer. There are also some children who develop cancer in early life who, if cured of the first cancer, are genetically prone to a second cancer in later life. This applies especially to some children with a cancer of the eye known as retinoblastoma. Only a minority of children with retinoblastoma have this propensity to a second cancer.

There are also some rare families with an unusually high incidence of cancer among adults and children. How this happens is not known. This situation usually comes to attention because two consecutive children or two closely related adults develop the same cancer.

In identical twins, if one develops acute lymphocytic leukemia, there is a 20% chance that the other will also develop the same type of leukemia within six months. Beyond six months the risk to the second twin is no greater than in the general population.

SUMMARY

The bulk of scientific evidence now suggests that childhood cancer is caused by a chance error in the formation or distribution of DNA during the phase of cell multiplication. There may be a wide variety of triggers which can set off such a cancer cell to multiply and cause the disease which is recognized as cancer. With rare exceptions, there are few environmental causes of childhood cancer.

CHAPTER 2

Incidence of Childhood Cancers

Children's cancers are rare, but occur in all parts of the world. They can occur in any race but some cancers are more common in some races and rare in others.

The best statistics on the frequency of childhood cancers are obtained from countries with large populations where large groups of children can be surveyed and where the incidence of cancer is assessed by registration of the diagnosis rather than death from cancer. Such a survey has been conducted in the USA and showed the following results, which are given as approximations (Table I).

REGIONAL VARIATION

The incidence of childhood cancer may vary from country to country but accurate information is difficult to obtain because it depends on the types of health system delivery, facilities for accurate diagnosis, and notification of diagnosis. In general, unlike the cancers of adults there is little variation in the incidence of childhood cancers from one country to another.

RACIAL VARIATION

Variation according to race is well documented. A cancer of the bones known as Ewing's sarcoma is very uncommon among the blacks of the USA. A cancer of the lymphatic tissues known as Burkitt's lymphoma is more common in African blacks than other races. It must be stressed however, that no race is exempt from childhood cancer.

CLUSTERS OF LEUKEMIA

The occurrence of an unexpectedly large number of people with the same disease in a certain geographic area is called a cluster. Occasionally such clusters of childhood leukemia have been reported in the USA, Australia and Britain. Thorough investigation has not established that these clusters may not have occurred by chance alone. No common factor involving life styles, geographic conditions or environmental factors have been dis-

TABLE 1

Incidence of childhood cancers.

Cancer	*Rate per 100,000 children under the age of 15 years*
Acute lymphocytic leukemia	3.0
Acute myeloid leukemia	0.5
Wilms tumor	0.8
Hodgkin's disease	0.8
Non-Hodgkin's lymphoma	1.4
Osteosarcoma	0.4
Ewings sarcoma	0.4
Rhabdomyosarcoma	0.4
Neuroblastoma	0.8
Unusual soft tissue tumors	0.3
Germ cell tumors of ovary or testis	0.2
Germ cell tumors of spinal origin	0.03
Brain tumors	2.5
Retinoblastoma	0.3
Histiocytosis X	0.2

covered between these various clusters. It is fair to conclude that clustering of leukemia occurs by chance alone.

SUMMARY

The chance of developing cancer in children under the age of 15 years is approximately 11/100 000 or 0.011 percent per year. The incidence varies little from one country to the next and no racial group is exempt.

CHAPTER 3

Treatment and Cure of Cancer

The majority of childhood cancers can be cured with intensive and often prolonged treatment in medical units which specialize in childhood cancer. These units are either situated in Children's Hospitals, or are a part of a comprehensive cancer treatment hospital. The treatment of a child with cancer is a team effort. The teams can be divided into the clinical and the laboratory teams. The clinical one usually consists of medical and surgical specialists in cancer treatment and younger doctors who are training to become such specialists, trained specialist nursing staff and their assistants, special pharmacists, medical social workers, clerical staff, physiotherapists, play therapists and occupational therapists, psychologists and psychiatrists and chaplains. The clinical team concept is illustrated in Figure 4. The laboratory team, which often works behind the scenes consists of scientific and medical staff who undertake tests in service and research laboratories. The results of the laboratory investigations are essential for the function of the clinical team.

GENERAL PRINCIPLES OF CANCER TREATMENT

The general principle is *cell kill!*

To kill all cancer cells one must know precisely what type of cancer it is, where it is situated in the body and where and how the cancer cells may have spread.

To establish the type of cancer, it is necessary to do some form of minor surgery or bone marrow testing. The specimen is then processed by scientists for microscopic examination and for a variety of specialized tests to accurately determine the type

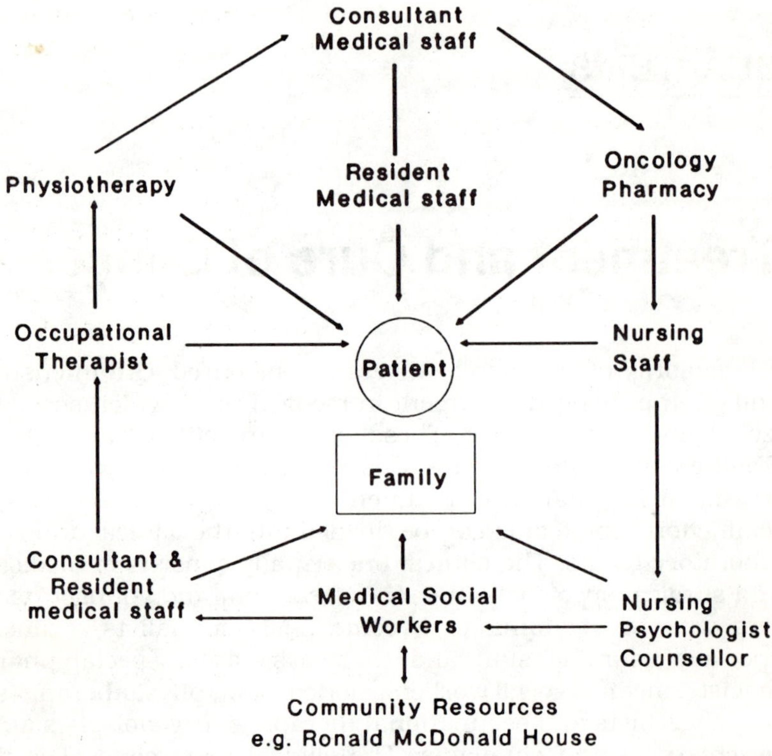

FIGURE 4 The clinical cancer treatment team.

of cancer and as many properties of the cancer as can be ascertained through the application of scientific research methods. Sometimes it may be necessary to wait some days before all the important information can be gathered. This delay very seldom has a bad effect on treatment and the old adage of "fools rush in where wise men fear to tread" is particularly applicable to this phase of waiting.

CANCER CELL SPREAD

The spread of cancer cells can take place by direct growth into adjoining tissues or organs or by growth in two types of vessels.

1. The lymphatic vessels which collect fluid from organs and pass this fluid along to lymph nodes. Eventually this fluids drains into the blood vessels.
2. Blood Vessels through which the blood circulates.

If the cancer cells enter the lymphatic vessels they lodge in lymph nodes where they can grow to a large size. They can also grow from one lymph node to another and in a stepwise fashion drain into the blood vessels. If the cancer cells enter the blood vessels they can circulate rapidly throughout the body and lodge and grow where there is a favorable environment for their growth. Spread of cancer by either of these routes gives rise to satellite cancers and this is called metastatic disease.

STAGING OF CANCER

The first step in treating cancer after it has been diagnosed and its type determined by the pathologists and scientists, is to find out how far it has spread. This is called *staging*. It can be compared to mapping the full extent and disposition of enemy forces. The staging process usually requires a variety of x-ray investigations, nuclear medicine and bone marrow tests. The x-ray investigations are usually plain x-rays, ultrasounds and CAT (computerized axial tomography) or MRI (magnetic resonance imaging) scans. The nuclear medicine techniques involve the injection of a small dose of a harmless radioactive material which is concentrated in certain tissues, such as bones in the presence of the cancer. The bone marrow aspirate or biopsy tests for the presence of the cancer cells in the marrow cavity. When all these tests are combined the extent of spread of the cancer can usually be assessed. However, only masses of cells 0.5cm or greater can be detected by these methods. There are no tests which can detect the presence of a few cancer cells only.

Surgical Staging

In some cases it is critical to know the spread of the tumor to lymph nodes with a precision which is even greater than that which can be obtained with CAT or, MRI scans or lymphangiography. Under such circumstances it is necessary to stage the cancer by undertaking surgery which is called a laparotomy.

This enables the surgeons to take small samples of organs and lymph nodes so that examination under a microscope can determine whether or not cancer cells have spread to these tissues.

Circumstances where Staging is not Required

The process of staging is performed in virtually all the cancers but details vary from one to another. The usual staging techniques will be dealt with under individual chapters on various forms of cancer. There are two important exceptions to this type of staging approach, and they are *leukemia* and *widespread neuroblastoma.* In the case of leukemia it is known that the disease is always widespread and the only question is whether it has spread to the central nervous system (brain and spinal cord). This can be tested for by a simple spinal tap (lumbar puncture) and occasionally a CAT scan of the brain. In some children with widespread neuroblastoma there is bone marrow involvement, and a bone marrow test, together with a urine test for the chemicals produced by the neuroblastoma, is all that is necessary for diagnosis and staging of the cancer.

In brain tumors the process of staging is also different because the important question is how far the tumor has spread within the central nervous system rather than outside of it. With rare exceptions brain tumors do not spread to organs outside the nervous system.

APPROACHES TO TREATMENT

Surgery

The simplest way of killing cancer cells is to remove them surgically. When the surgeons operate for cancer they use some form of a knife to remove lumps of cancer cells. Surgeons however cannot see individual cells and their instruments cannot separate cells. In order to remove as much as possible of the cancer the surgeons plan the operation in such a way as to remove adjoining tissues which may have been infiltrated by the cancer cells. This margin of normal tissues that may have to be removed varies from one body organ to another. Occasionally the anatomical situation of the cancer forces one to remove a whole organ such as the kidney or to amputate a limb.

In childhood cancer surgical removal of the main cancer site is usually the most desirable approach in dealing with the bulk of the cancer because, in the long term, surgery has the least number of undesirable long term consequences. There are however certain instances where surgery cannot be used because of the severe mutilation that it would cause, as for example in tumors of the pelvis, or the head and neck regions.

Limitations of Surgery

Unfortunately in the majority of patients surgery alone cannot cure the cancer. The reasons for surgical failure are the inability of the surgery to remove all cancer cells at the local site of the origin of the cancer as well as its inability to deal with the spread of cancer cells to distant parts of the body.

Chemotherapy

The major advance which has resulted in cures of childhood cancer is the use of chemotherapy. Chemotherapy means chemical treatment. In the case of cancer, chemotherapy is aimed at the *killing of cells*. The concept of cancer chemotherapy is similar to the use of antibiotics to treat infections but there is an essential difference. Antibiotics kill foreign organisms but not the body's cells. Chemotherapy kills not only cancer cells but also those cells of the body which retain an ability to multiply. These are the cells of the bone marrow, the gut, hair follicles and in some cases those of the reproductive organs e.g. the testes. Chemotherapy does not kill the cells of the body which normally do not multiply e.g. brain, lung, heart or kidney cells.

The killing of cells that retain the ability to multiply is the reason that chemotherapy is effective in curing childhood cancers. It is also the reason for the toxic effects of chemotherapy. These two effects are inseparable because cancer cells, unlike bacteria or other foreign organisms, do not differ substantially from the normal cells of the body.

Chemotherapy can cure certain cancers for 2 main reasons:

1. Cancer cells multiply more slowly than normal cells. Therefore normal cells can recover more rapidly from the killing effect of chemotherapy than do cancer cells. Repeated use of chemotherapy over a period will therefore lead to total or near total cancer cell kill without extermination of normal cells. This concept is illustrated in Figure 5.
2. There are subtle biochemical differences between certain cancer cells and normal cells and these differences can be used to select chemotherapy which will have special advantages in killing cancer cells.

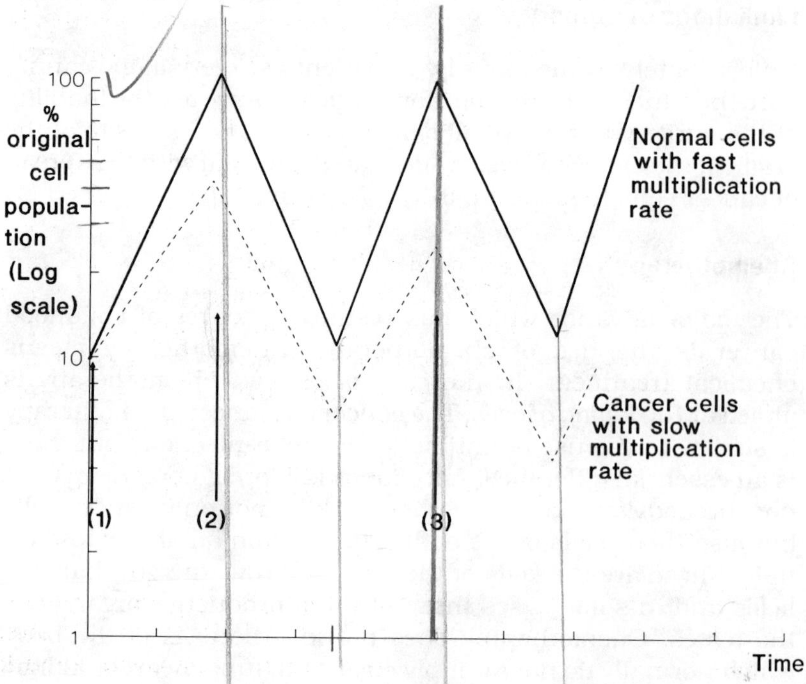

FIGURE 5 Preferential kill of cancer cells by chemotherapy. The first dose of chemotherapy (1) kills 90% of normal and cancer cells. The normal cells multiply more rapidly than the cancer cells. By the time the second dose of chemotherapy (2) is given, normal cells have recovered to 100% but cancer cells to only 50%. When chemotherapy is repeated (3) there is a stepwise reduction of cancer cells without a similar reduction of normal cells.

Limitations of Chemotherapy

Apart from the toxic effects of chemotherapy on normal cells there are other drawbacks.

1. Sanctuaries

   Effective levels of chemotherapeutic agents which will kill cancer cells can only be achieved in areas of the body where there is a good circulation and the drugs can get out of the blood stream into the fluid surrounding the cancer cells.

   There are certain parts of the body where this is not possible, or the process is inefficient. These parts include the brain, eyes, testes and bones and these are called sanctuary sites.

2. Drug Resistance

   Another problem with chemotherapy is the development of resistance to the killing effects of the drugs. All chemotherapeutic agents kill multiplying cells by damaging the production, organization and repair of the inheritance material—DNA. Cells can develop alternate ways to prevent or to repair the damage caused by chemotherapy. Such cells have a growth advantage over the cells which are damaged by chemotherapy and this leads to overgrowth of drug resistant cells. This problem with chemotherapy can, to a considerable degree be overcome, by using combinations of chemotherapeutic agents at the biggest dose that the patient can tolerate.

3. Long Term Complications

   Since chemotherapy acts by damaging the DNA it has the potential to cause changes in the DNA which may in later years cause cancer. So far only one type of chemotherapeutic agent, known as alkylating agents, have been shown to cause second late cancers in a small number of individuals.

Chemotherapy: the Breakthrough in Cancer Treatment

Despite these drawbacks the appropriate use of chemotherapy has been the cause of the major breakthrough in the cure of childhood cancer. Development of new agents and studies of their usefulness in childhood cancer have saved many thousands of lives. Effective treatment of childhood cancer without chemotherapy is only seldom possible. In the years prior to chemotherapy, no more than 5–10% of children with cancer were cured. In the 1980s the overall cure rates are 70%.

Radiation Therapy

The third modality of childhood cancer treatment is the use of radiation therapy, or what is commonly called x-ray therapy. Like surgery, radiation therapy can effectively deal with a local cancer but not with sites of spread of the cancer by lymph or blood vessels. Radiation therapy is most effective in eradicating cancer when the cancers are small rather than large. It is often most effective in ensuring total cancer cell kill at the local site of the cancer's growth after the bulk of the cancer has been decreased by surgery or chemotherapy.

Limitation of Radiation Therapy

Unfortunately, in children, radiation therapy has some serious long term consequences. The major characteristics of childhood are growth and development. Muscles, bones and all other organs grow during childhood to achieve adult size. Radiation therapy arrests or slows the growth of normal cells at the site where the radiation has been given. In time this leads to deformities of the body which have serious cosmetic, and therefore psychological consequences. The lack of growth of the irradiated tissues can also markedly interfere with their function. This can be particularly troublesome when large doses of radiation have to be used in treating the brain, lungs or the heart.

Like chemotherapy, radiation therapy kills cancer cells by damaging DNA. It therefore can have side effects by killing normal multiplying cells such as those in the bone marrow and gut. It can also damage the DNA in such a way that a second later cancer can occur.

Role of Radiation Therapy

Despite these disadvantages radiation therapy does have a significant role in the treatment of childhood cancer. It is the only way to ensure good local control of cancer cells which have or may have spread to adjoining organs that cannot be surgically excised e.g. from the kidney to the liver. It can kill cells in sanctuary sites which are otherwise protected from chemotherapy e.g. leukemia cells in the brain. It can also control the rate of growth of cancer cells in sites of the body which cannot be operated upon or where surgery and chemotherapy have failed and there is regrowth of the tumor causing pain or compression of vital organs. The form of treatment in which radiation therapy is used to control symptoms rather than cure the patient is known as palliative.

SUMMARY OF STRATEGIES OF TREATMENT

In this chapter a number of complicated concepts and strategies have been introduced. They can be summarized as follows:

1. Most childhood cancers can be cured.
2. The treatment is complicated and protracted.
3. The first step in treatment is diagnosis of the type of tumor and its staging.
4. Surgery may play a major role in removing the bulk of tumor but on its own is seldom curative.
5. Chemotherapy is the principal modality of anti-cancer treatment and is the major way of killing all cancer cells.
6. Radiation therapy has a well defined but limited role in the treatment of childhood cancers.

CURE RATES OF THE MAJOR CHILDHOOD CANCERS

The percentage of cures in these cancers is based on experience reported by major cancer treatment centers. Cure is defined as a state of health where the chance of dying as a result of a recurrence of the cancer is not significantly greater than in the non-cancer affected population. Cure rates in the variety of childhood cancers is shown in Table II.

TABLE 2
The rates of cure in childhood cancer.

Cancer		*Estimated cure rate*
Acute lymphocytic leukemia		75%
Acute Myeloid leukemia		60%
Wilms' tumor		90+%
Hodgkin's disease		90+%
Non Hodgkin's lymphoma		60–70%
Osteosarcoma		70%
Ewings sarcoma		50%
Rhabdomyosarcoma	early stage	90%
	late stage	20%
Neuroblastoma	early stage	90+%
	late stage	5%
Unusual soft tissue tumors		60%
Germ cell tumors of ovary or testes		80%
Germ cell tumors of spinal column origin		70%
Brain tumors		40%
Retinoblastomas		90%

CHAPTER 4

Tests and Procedures in Childhood Cancer

During the process of diagnosis, staging and treatment of the cancer, a number of technical procedures which require needles and injections must be performed. When the skin of the child has to be breached with a needle it produces fear and pain. It is an invasive procedure!!

The boundary between the internal environment and the outside is skin. The nerve supply of the skin is rich, and sensations from the skin are registered in the sensory parts of the brain. A breach of this barrier is naturally frightening and painful. The parents, doctors and nurses attending the child with cancer can diminish the shock of breech of the integrity of the body by reducing the element of fear, but unfortunately it is not possible to fully remove the feeling of anticipation and pain.

The key to removal of fear of the procedure is to have one or both parents of the child present when the procedure is being undertaken, and for them to show the child that they understand why the procedure is being undertaken and that they are not afraid of it. The parents have to try to keep a perspective on the transient and relatively minor discomfort of a procedure when compared to its possible benefits. It is important to neither exaggerate or minimize the child's apprehension and pain. By all means sympathise with the child but keep these feelings in perspective.

Co-operative behavior by the child during a procedure should be rewarded by appropriate praise or even gifts from the parent. Bad behavior should be ignored. It is important to pay as little attention as possible to "naughty" behavior and to persist with the procedure so that the child learns that bad behavior will not be rewarded by postponement or even abandonment of the procedure.

Professional staff performing or assisting with procedures should be friendly and considerate and explain them in plain language. Preparations for the procedure which are time consuming and do not require the presence of the patient should be undertaken in the patient's absence. If at all possible the procedure should be performed as quickly as possible and the staff should thank the patient for their cooperation.

Inevitably there will be occasions where through technical difficulty, the first or second attempts at a procedure fail.At such times it is often better to abandon the procedure and repeat it at another time when the patient, family members and staff have recovered from the variety of aggressive and guilt feelings which are associated with a failed procedure. There is no shame in requesting that a difficult procedure be undertaken by a more experienced staff member.

PRE-MEDICATION

Medications to reduce pain and anxiety of procedures are often known as "pre-meds". These usually consist of an intramuscular injection of morphine or one of its derivatives, together with a drug that induces drowsiness and a temporary loss of memory. In theory this is a good way to reduce the unpleasantness of technical procedures but in practice it means that the child has an extra injection, which is also painful. In general, most children prefer to have no pre-medication for procedures, and whenever possible after having become familiar with the procedures, should be allowed to have their choice.

There are still some centers where procedures such as bone marrow aspirates and spinal taps are undertaken under a short lasting general anesthetic. In rare instances children may have a severe fear of procedures which requires the use of general anesthesia, but mostly the risks of a general anesthetic are not worth taking for these relatively minor procedures.

OTHER MEANS OF ALLEVIATING PAIN OF PROCEDURES

Hypnosis, music therapy and psychological counselling are being used in some centers to reduce anxiety and pain of procedures. Their success depends largely on the skills of the operator and the cooperation of the child and family. Where such services are available they may prove to be useful to a variable proportion of children.

ANTI-EMETICS

Chemotherapy is often associated with nausea and vomiting and many children and adults find this to be one of its most unpleasant consequences. Chemotherapy induces vomiting by a direct effect on chemicals produced in the gastrointestinal tract and possibly by irritation of the vomiting center in the brain stem. A complete understanding on how chemotherapy causes vomiting is lacking. To prevent or reduce vomiting most cancer treatment centers have developed their own anti-emetic drug combinations. Recently a very promising new drug has been developed which may stop or reduce vomiting with chemotherapy, without inducing drowsiness.

In general, drugs which prevent vomiting are given prior to, or with the injection of the chemotherapeutic agent, and usually in addition to reduction of vomiting cause drowsiness. Drugs which have to be given by mouth in nauseated or vomiting children are seldom effective because they are soon vomited.

There is some evidence that smoking of cannabis or taking it by mouth may reduce the nausea and vomiting of certain forms of chemotherapy but controlled studies have shown cannabis to be only minimally superior to more conventional agents.

Anticipatory Vomiting

This occurs in some children and is characterized by vomiting on the way to, or soon after arrival at, the treatment center. It is not an indication of a psychological disturbance but simply a variant of the chemically induced vomiting. In such children the anxiety associated with chemotherapy induces a release of vomiting inducing chemicals. Paradoxically, once these children have vomited they tolerate their chemotherapy well and usually do not vomit much after chemotherapy is finished. There are no adequate drugs to prevent "anticipatory vomiting" and attempts at psychological and conditioning treatments only further embarrass the child and their family.

BONE MARROW ASPIRATE

In certain bones of the body such as the hip bones there is active production of bone marrow. The bone marrow is made in the soft center of the bone and is contained by outer layers of compact or hard bone. A bone marrow aspirate consists of insertion of a needle through the compact outer layer into the spongy soft bone and suction of a sample of the bone marrow. This is illustrated diagramatically in Figure 6 and a photograph of the usual equipment is shown in Figure 7.

The usual places for a bone marrow aspirate are the top of the hip bones, at either the front or the back near the spine. The aspirate can be performed with either a special bone marrow needle which is rather thick, or with a thinner spinal tap needle.

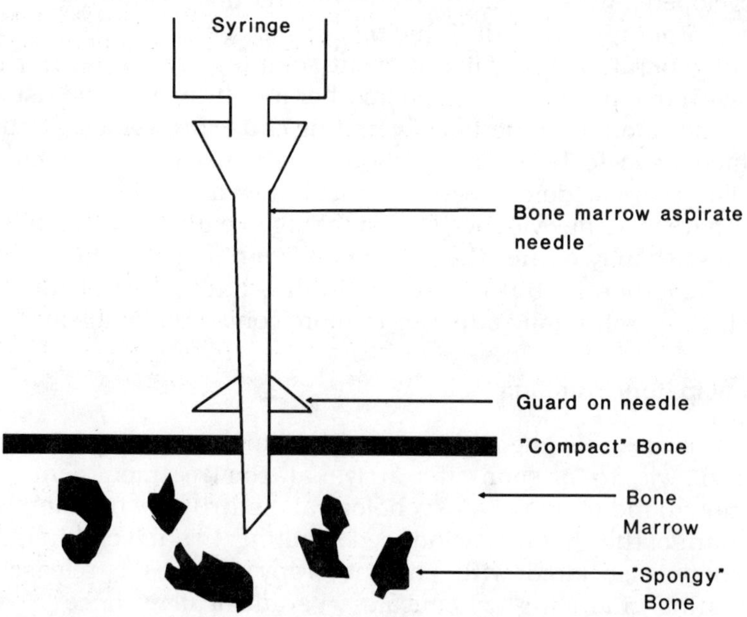

FIGURE 6 Diagramatic representation of bone marrow aspirate.

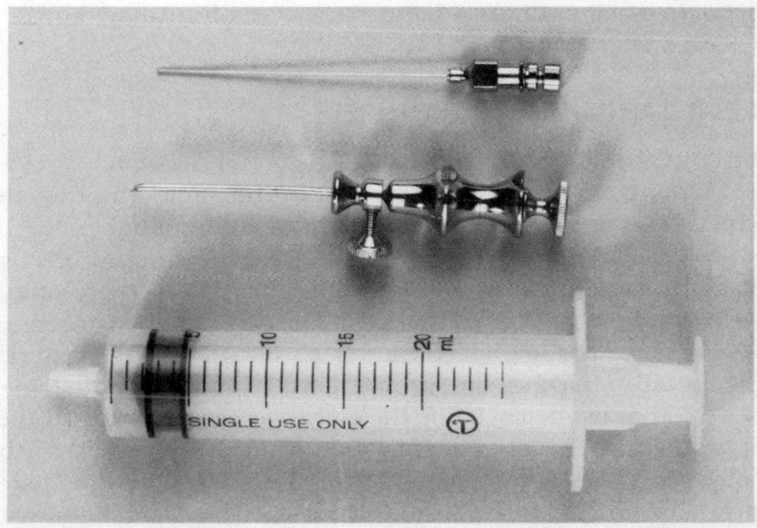

FIGURE 7 Bone marrow aspirate needle next to the syringe used for aspirating the marrow. The top screw in the needle is part of the stilette while the bottom screw is part of the guard. Above the bone marrow aspirate needle is a spinal tap needle which under some circumstances can also be used for bone marrow aspiration.

Pain with the aspirate is due to the needle penetrating skin, muscle and tissue planes near the outer compact layer of bone. In addition pain is also produced by suction of the bone marrow. The pain produced by penetrating skin and tissue planes can be abolished by a skin anesthetic cream and by injection of local anesthetic in the same way as with dental procedures. The pain of suction is not preventable but is only momentary.

Bone Marrow Trephine

This is a similar procedure to an aspirate but in this case rather than sucking out marrow a piece of soft internal part of the bone is cut out. To accomplish this one needs a wide bore needle and its insertion into the bone is much more painful. To alleviate this pain it is wise to use pre-medication as well as a local anesthetic. In some patients a bone marrow trephine may require a general anesthetic.

SPINAL TAP (LUMBAR PUNCTURE)

The spine consists of bones called the vertebrae which enclose the spinal cord and the nerve roots in the same way that the skull encloses the brain. Within the spinal column and the skull, the spinal cord and brain are surrounded by protective membranes, and bathed in a fluid called the cerebro-spinal fluid which is abbreviated to "CSF". The vertebral bones consist of an anterior portion called the vertebral body, and a posterior portion called the vertebral arch. The vertebral bodies are joined to each other by "discs" while the arches are joined to each other by ligaments. These ligaments are relatively soft and can be easily penetrated by a sharp needle. A spinal tap is the insertion of such a fine needle through the ligaments and membranes surrounding the cord at a part of the lower back where the spinal cord has finished and only its nerve roots are present in the spinal canal. The hollow needle allows the CSF to be collected for laboratory examination and can be used for injection of selected chemotherapeutic agents directly into the CSF. This is diagramatically illustrated in Figures 8 and 9. The spinal tap procedure is photographed in Figure 10.

In small children the back is flexible and the spinal tap is usually not very painful. In general no premedication is required. In adolescents a spinal tap may be followed by headache which is thought to be due to alterations of pressure between the skull and lower part of the spinal column. This headache can often be prevented by lying the patient flat on their back for 24 hours following the spinal tap. Pre-medication and anesthetics do not prevent the post spinal tap headache. Where post spinal tap headache is a disabling symptom admission to a hospital for 24 hours may be required with each spinal tap.

OMMAYA AND RICKHAM RESERVOIRS

In some children where spinal taps prove to be exceedingly difficult, and occasionally for other medical reasons, it may be necessary to introduce a device which is anchored in the skull

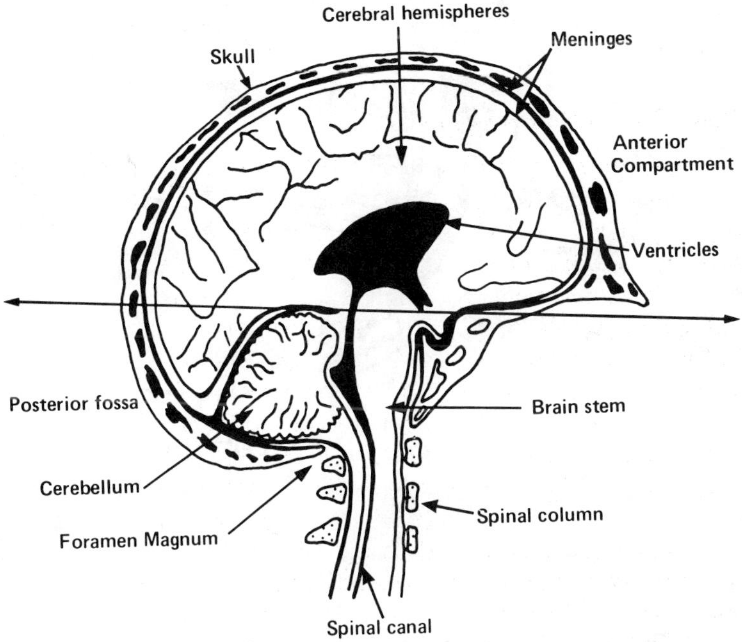

FIGURE 8 Brain and the top of the spinal cord enclosed within the skull and spinal column. The cerebrospinal fluid bathes the brain and spinal cord and circulates through the ventricles and the spinal canal.

and which has a thin catheter that sits inside fluid containing cavities of the brain known as ventricles (Figure 8). These devices are inserted by neurosurgeons with the patient under general anesthesia and can be used to sample CSF, and introduce drugs into the CSF. In children with brain tumors these devices are used to reduce the build-up of pressure in the brain caused by a blockage of the circulation of CSF by the tumor. This build-up of pressure is known as raised intra-cranial pressure, and it causes hydrocephalus.

In general it is preferable to administer drugs into the CSF by a spinal tap rather than into the reservoirs, because of the possibility of infection of the reservoir.

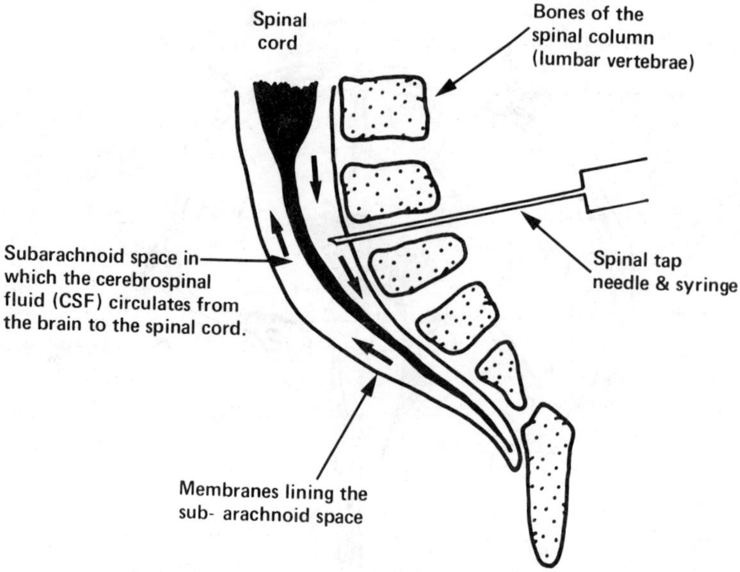

FIGURE 9 Spinal cord and the spinal tap.

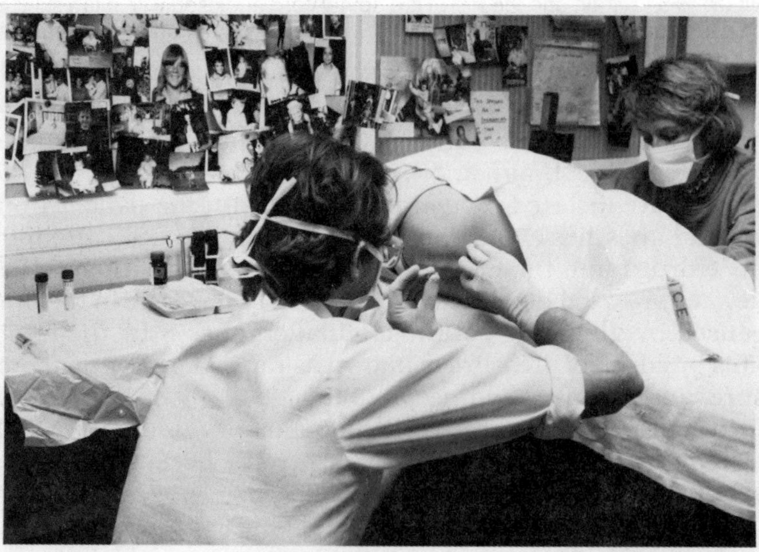

FIGURE 10 Performing a spinal tap.

INTRAVENOUS NEEDLES, LINES AND CATHETERS

The great majority of substances used to treat cancer have to be administered directly into the blood stream. This can best be done by inserting some device into the vein and this is called a venepuncture.

For the majority of children there are a number of commercially manufactured intravenous needles, with or without external plastic catheters, which can be inserted through the skin directly into the vein with only moderate discomfort. Appropriate local anesthetic creams applied at the site of the venepuncture can reduce the pain of skin penetration. Efficient insertion of needles and careful maintenance by a skilled person are details of management which are readily overlooked when all goes well, but become almost insurmountable obstacles if there are persistent difficulties.

Recently there have been very satisfactory new developments which have helped to overcome problems associated with difficult venous access. These devices are in principle similar to the Ommaya and Rickham reservoirs used for access into the CSF. They are essentially of two types.

1. The Hickman or Broviac catheters are lines which penetrate the skin and then are tunnelled under the skin along the chest wall to a major blood vessel in the neck, and thence inside the blood vessel to just above the heart (Figure 11). Because one end of the lines penetrates the skin they can become infected. They must therefore be handled in a sterile manner. Special dressings are required and the outlets of these lines are in one way or another anchored to the skin of the chest wall. The advantages of these lines are that they are multichannelled, thereby permitting simultaneous introduction of different treatment agents e.g. blood products, antibiotics and chemotherapy.
2. The infusaport or portacaths work on a similar principle but they do not penetrate the skin. Instead a reservoir is inserted under the skin and surgically anchored to the surrounding tissues (Figure 12). Since the reservoir is under the skin the risk of infection is greatly reduced as is the inconvenience of regular dressings. Their disadvantage is that they only have

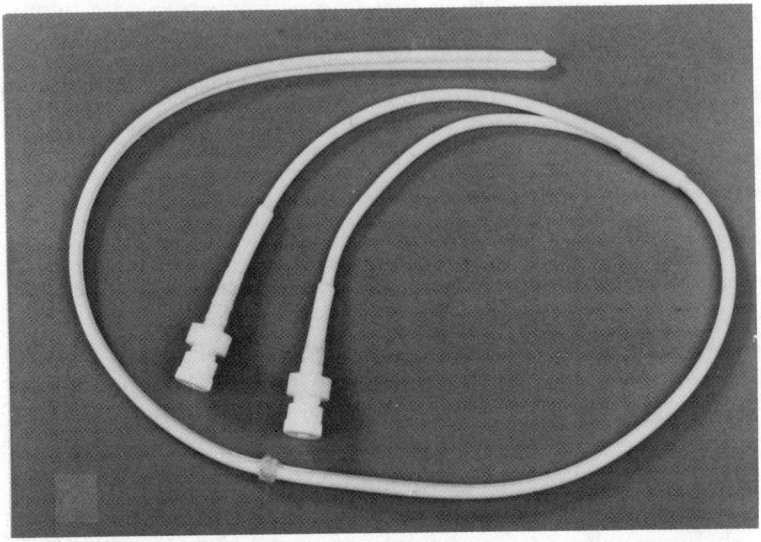

FIGURE 11 Double lumen Hickman catheter.

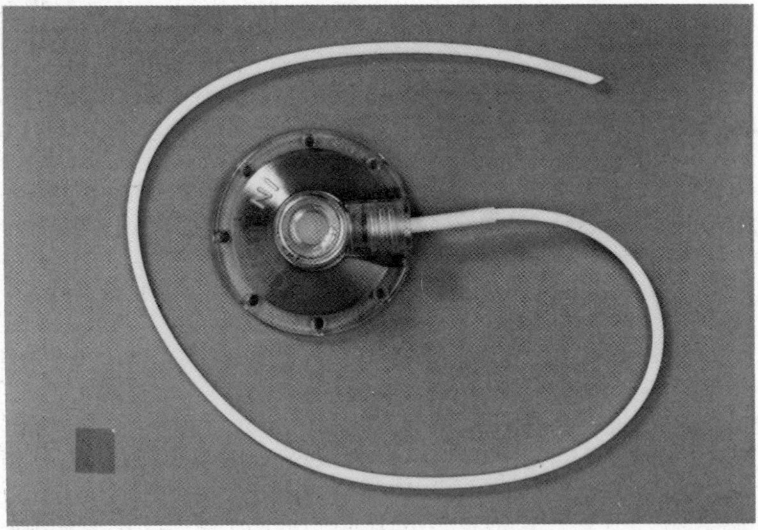

FIGURE 12 Infusaport. The reservoir is inserted under the skin and can be entered by a special needle through a sealed opening at the top of the reservoir.

a single channel and that each time they are used a needle has to be inserted through the skin into the reservoir.

In general Hickman or Broviac catheters are preferred in patients likely to require extensive procedures such as bone marrow transplant. In most other patients where venous access is a significant problem a reservoir situated under the skin is the device of choice. These intravenous devices are shown in Figure 11.

RADIOLOGIC PROCEDURES

During the course of investigation, staging and treatment of childhood cancer, some or many radiologic investigations will

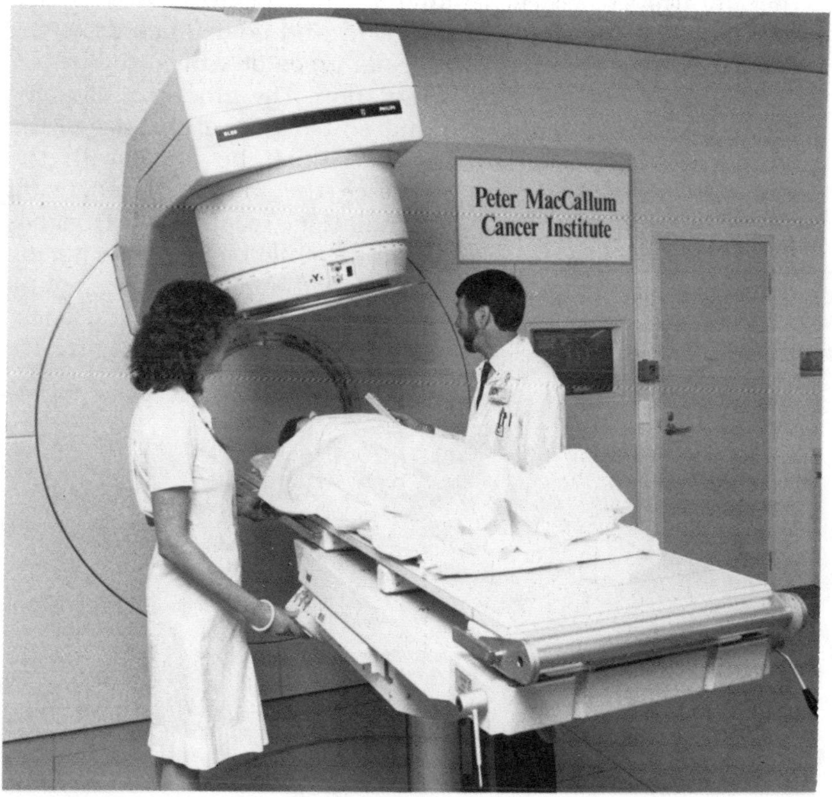

FIGURE 13 Equipment used for irradiation.

be required. They are not painful but may be frightening because of the size and the presentation of the machinery. In addition, for these investigations the child may be required to be immobile for prolonged periods of time. Whenever possible it is preferable to use sedation to obtain immobility for investigations, but in small children general anesthesia may be required. It is safer to administer a general anesthetic under the control of an anesthetist than to give large doses of sedatives which can depress respiration.

RADIATION THERAPY

This is given by means of a variety of machines which are housed in reserved areas of a hospital or in special radiation therapy units. Prior to irradiation the doctors and radiation physicists plan the irradiation field and sometimes draw the fields on the patients skin. Special types of x-rays may be required to plan the fields of irradiation. The procedure is painless but it is frightening to children because of the size of the equipment and because the child must be alone with the machine for a few minutes. Once the initial apprehension diminishes children do not fear radiation. To administer irradiation effectively it is important that the child be immobile during delivery of the irradiation. To ensure that this occurs young children may require sedation, and rarely, even general anesthesia. The appearance of the equipment is shown in Figure 13.

CHAPTER 5

Responses and Emotions at the Time of Diagnosis

People are different, and their response to devastating news also differs in detail. Nevertheless, this response has certain definable phases. It is helpful to be able to recognize these, as this can help to make adjustments in the way of life, which are necessary when caring for a child with cancer.

DISBELIEF AND SHOCK

The earliest phase is one of disbelief and shock. The words used by the doctor do not truly enter the consciousness of the parents or guardians, and when they do, it feels as if they did not apply to their child. The time gap between being given the information and registering the appropriate response to it varies with different circumstances. If a family doctor warned the family of the likelihood of a diagnosis of cancer, the time of shock and disbelief after confirmation of the diagnosis is often short. If the diagnosis is given without any preparation, then the duration of shock and disbelief may be long. The initial interview with the doctor is also particularly important because it establishes the first bonds between the family and the doctor and allied health professionals present at the interview. This bond forms the basis of a relationship of trust and therefore confidence in the decision making process regarding treatment.

Often during this interview the doctor discusses details of the likely outcome of treatment and details of the type of treatment. Usually, it is difficult for the family at this interview to understand and remember all that they have been told. It is important to remember that there will be other opportunities for further interviews which will give the chance to ask questions and clarify details which may have been forgotten.

At times there are strong feelings of unreality by one or other parent during the initial interview. They may involve disbelief of the diagnosis and the wish for other medical opinions. While this is usually unnecessary it is often better to be convinced than have a lingering doubt about the correctness of the diagnosis. In such cases a second opinion is warranted provided that it can be rapidly obtained. Third, fourth and fifth opinions are usually counterproductive and lead to alienation between the family and the treatment team.

Another not uncommon emotion at the time of diagnosis is anger, sometimes accompanied by fantasies of violence. This may be directed at other people or occasionally at oneself. Some degree of anger at the injustice of the situation is normal, but in general, anger feelings at a time when the family requires the maximum support from friends and society are destructive. Feelings of anger do not help the child to cope with their illness or with the treatment that may be required.

ADJUSTMENT

The phase of shock and disbelief is followed by adjustment to the diagnosis and changes of life style which are inevitably associated with cancer treatment. In the earliest phases of adjustment some degree of depression is common. There is a loss of interest in family, friends and recreational activities. All attention is focussed on the child and the treatment of the disease. Sometimes this phase is followed by one of euphoria in which everything seems to be proceeding better than average and each small item of good information about the response to treatment is given exaggerated importance. This often stems from anxiety and a need for reassurance to reduce the anxiety.

After some weeks the adjustment process reaches stability, with a reshaping of the family's life style to fit in with the diagnosis and treatment of the disease. This life style is usually very different from that before the onset of the illness. It is often more inwardly oriented, centered on the ill child and the home environment, less concerned with future planning and the external trappings of success. Frequently both parents give up some or many of their external commitments and this may mean financial and career sacrifices.

As time passes by without recurrence of cancer there is a gradual return to the family's previous life style until, with the passage of many years, the disease becomes a memory of a major past event rather than an ever present anxiety.

PROBLEMS OF ADJUSTING

Many problems can occur during the adjustment phase. The stress of the child's illness will test the relationship of the parents. Pre-existing stresses are usually exacerbated and subconscious feelings of anger and resentment by one or other parent may surface and cause a rift in the family. One essential and practical means of preventing these problems is for both parents to be involved in the care of the child and dealings with staff, not only while in hospital, but also when receiving treatment from home. Such a "team" effort allows both parents to understand the problems and frustrations of the details of treatment and avoids misunderstandings that can lead to family arguments.

SIBLING REACTIONS

The siblings of the ill child often feel neglected because the attention of all the family is focussed on the sick child. This is a natural reaction of children and not a callous attitude. Explanations of the reasons for apparent neglect are usually only temporarily helpful. One of the best ways to reduce sibling jealousy is to encourage them to visit the sick child in hospital not only when things are going well but also when they are going badly. Witnessing nausea and vomiting, episodes of high fever and hair loss soon eliminates jealous feelings by the healthy sibling and fosters their natural sympathy for the sick child. It is more effective than words in explaining why the parents are concentrating on their ill child.

PATERNAL ESCAPISM

Not all parents can cope in the same way and to the same degree, with the stress of a potentially fatal illness. Each parent has their individual strengths and weaknesses. Sometimes a parent, most often the father, will use work or financial circumstances to escape from the stress of shared responsibility for the child's treatment. Most often this manifests itself by giving work commitments a higher priority than being with the sick child and it can progress to a form of escapism where work consumes almost all of the father's time. The care of the sick child is delegated to the mother with the father becoming an interested bystander who nevertheless reserves for himself the right to make important decisions. This pattern of behavior is fraught with danger for the whole family and not infrequently leads to separation of the parents.

MATERNAL ESCAPISM

This is far less frequent and almost unknown in the early phases of adjustment. When it occurs, it manifests itself by excessive involvement of the maternal grandmother in the child's care, to the extent that the grandmother takes responsibility for most of the home and hospital care. The mother withdraws by becoming increasingly helpless with even such tasks as arrangements for transport or meals. The father of the child who may wish to step in and assist is often pushed aside by mother and grandmother and declared to be too busy or to be incompetent. As with paternal escapism this is also a destructive reaction which leads to family breakdown.

DEPRESSION

As previously mentioned one or other, less often both parents, can experience a prolonged and sometimes severe period of depression. This usually affects them gradually and manifests itself by a pronounced and sustained fall in the standard of home meals and hygiene; running down of the maintenance standards of their dwelling; untidy appearance; failure to keep appointments; poor compliance with medications; excessive dependence on sedatives, cigarettes or alcohol; neglect of the healthy siblings and a fall in the family income due to poor work performance. These symptoms, manifesting themselves to a minor degree, are very common, but if they are major features of the family's life and are prolonged, then they require professional intervention by medical social workers; psychologists or psychiatrists.

SEARCH FOR "MAGIC CURES"

Another manifestation of denial and depression is the search for "magic" cures. This usually manifests itself as a disillusionment with the probabilities of cure offered by scientific medicine and the search for "alternative" treatment. Since scientific medicine can only offer probabilities of cure but not certainties many people long for something which will guarantee them a cure. This is a normal and wholly understandable wish, but unfortunately it is unrealistic. There are people and organizations in all communities that are prepared to cater for this need by using one or other so called "natural" treatment which they can guarantee not to harm the patient, and which in subtle terms is said to be good for the patient. Often these people will suggest that standard methods of medical treatment are continued, but that in addition, their treatment also be used. The major reason why they are attractive to some parents of children with cancer is that they give these parents some control over the actual weapons of treatment of cancer. The cure of the cancer of their child is not left only to the doctor and nurses. This is an understandable feeling but it can be harmful because it substitutes for love and care compliance with a diet or other forms of "natural" medication. The role of "alternative medicine" is fully discussed in Chapter 8.

EXPLAINING THE ILLNESS TO THE CHILD

The treatment of cancer in children is complicated and time consuming. One cannot expect any person to tolerate and endure such treatment without understanding the need for it. The difficulty with children is to construct an explanation of the disease which is appropriate to the age, intelligence and emotional maturity of the child.

There are some guidelines which can be applied in all situations.

1. The parents should be the first to inform the child about the disease.
2. The disease should be called by its proper name e.g. leukemia, Hodgkin's disease, osteosarcoma etc.
3. The child should be told that with treatment there is a good chance of getting rid of the disease, but that treatment will take a long time.
4. Only the early phases of treatment should be detailed rather than going over all the different stages of treatment.
5. No statements should be made about failure of treatment or the chances of death from the disease or the treatment.
6. The child should not be burdened with the possible complications of treatment until they are ready to ask about them.

The approach to each child will differ, and in adolescents the information may need to be given in more explicit language, but the principles remain the same. Above all, one must avoid deluging the adolescent with information that they do not wish to hear. On the other hand, questions should be answered as truthfully as possible.

In rare instances the patient may ask the question "will I die". The appropriate response to this question is to say that the treatment that they are about to receive is aimed at their cure and has a good chance of working and while there is some chance of death with treatment, there is a far greater chance of cure.

While it is the parents role to impart the initial information it will be reinforced and expanded by the professional staff in the treatment unit. This is done by personal discussion between the child and health professionals and also during ward rounds and bedside conferences which, in some instances, are meant not only for the teaching of staff, but also the parents and the patient.

EXPLAINING CANCER TO YOUNG CHILDREN

The details of how to do this will depend on the cultural context of the society that one lives in, as well as the current fashion in popular childhood stories. The general principle is to select a bad character that the child recognizes as being bad and who is engaged in battles with good characters, and to say that the child's body has been invaded by their disease in the same way as the bad character invades the good character's territory. The bad character is called "leukemia" or "lymphoma" etc. The good characters are the resistance of the child's body and their weapons are the treatment modalities that will be used in the treatment of the particular illness e.g. chemotherapy, surgery. Time will be required to conquer the illness but there will eventually be a victory. The last statement may in some instances be dishonest, but it is nevertheless desirable to preserve hope, for without it the child will not cooperate with treatment.

In addition to this type of explanation one should also introduce pleasant things to look forward to for the child at the completion of certain milestones in the course of treatment. If holidays or school camps have to be abandoned the child should be given firm prospects of subsequent pleasant alternatives.

Information at Relapse

The process described above applies to the time of the initial diagnosis. Should relapse occur a different method of discussion of information is required. This will be dealt with in the next chapter.

CHAPTER 6

Relapse

The term means that there has been a recurrence of the primary tumor either at its original site of presentation (local relapse/recurrence), or at distant sites (metastases). It is the most dreaded consequence of failure of cancer treatment, because with few exceptions, it means that cure from cancer is only a remote possibility. The exceptions to this pessimistic statement are:

1. isolated extramedullary relapses in acute leukemia,
2. relapse in Hodgkin's disease,
3. isolated lung metastases after discontinuation of treatment for solid tumors, particularly Wilms' tumor.

CAUSES OF RELAPSE

Sanctuaries

The occurrence of relapse essentially indicates a failure to eradicate all the cancer cells by whatever were the methods of treatment. This may be due to cancer cells being hidden in sanctuary sites where they are protected from the lethal effects of chemotherapy. Such sanctuary sites are:

1. central nervous system where the circulation comes into contact with a "fat barrier" (blood-brain barrier) which prevents the passage of drugs from the circulation to the tissues;
2. the eye where a similar situation pertains;
3. the testes where the mechanism is unknown;

4. other sites where the tumor cells are poorly supplied by blood vessels, e.g. bone.

Drug Resistance

Drug resistance implies that some cancer cells possess or develop mechanisms which can prevent, or rapidly repair, the damage to DNA which is caused by all anti-cancer agents. Such cells are most likely to exist when the tumor has been present in the patient for a long time, and when the tumor is very bulky. This is because cancer cells are genetically unstable, and have a higher rate of mutation than normal cells. The longer the tumor has been present, or the more cells there are (bulky tumor), the higher the chance of a mutation which can result in drug resistance. The emergence of drug resistance can be accelerated by ineffective early anti-cancer treatment which kills only the most sensitive cells, but leaves the resistant cells untouched. Under these circumstances the resistant cells have no environmental competition for nutrition and growth factors, and therefore multiply more rapidly. Most tumors have been present for a considerable time and even small tumors contain millions of cells. Therefore, there is a considerable chance that mutants resistant to certain pathways of drug induced-DNA damage, are present at the time of initial clinical presentation, in the majority of patients. It is unlikely however that these mutants have developed mechanisms to by-pass all the possible different pathways of inflicting DNA damage. It follows that the most effective anti-cancer therapy will consist of multiple drugs which have different mechanisms of causing DNA damage, given in their maximum tolerable dose. This principle of treatment is called the Goldie and Coldman hypothesis and is widely practised in modern oncology.

DIAGNOSIS OF RELAPSE

The frequent review visits by patients having cancer treatment are aimed at monitoring response to therapy, the side effects of the disease and its treatment, and whether there is evidence of relapse. Follow up tests such as blood count, x-rays and other special radiologic techniques are aimed at diagnosis of relapse as early as possible.

When a relapse is suspected it is usually necessary to undertake investigations to see whether it is isolated or widespread. In the case of leukemia this will require a bone marrow aspirate and a spinal tap. In the case of solid tumors a variety of special x-rays and radio-isotope scan may be required as well as a surgical biopsy to see the microscopic features of the relapsed tumor. All of these investigations are essential for making decisions on treatment with the first relapse but in 2nd, 3rd and later relapse they are seldom required.

TREATMENT OF RELAPSE

This depends on the nature of the tumor and is discussed in the chapters on individual tumors. The treatment of all types of relapses however, has one feature in common. The statement that a relapse has occurred is a sentence of death for the majority of patients. In modern oncology it is the time at which many parents, families and children are forced to confront early death.

IMPARTING THE NEWS OF RELAPSE

It is often best to do this in a gradual fashion by alerting the patient and family that further tests are required to establish the presence, and the possible extent of the relapse. This approach allows the family and the patient to consider over a period of time their response to the possibility of a relapse, and it allows the doctor and the treatment team to consider treatment options in a unhurried manner. There is little to be gained from informing the patient and family instantly of the presence of relapse, because immediate treatment of a relapse does not improve its prognosis.

EMOTIONAL RESPONSES

These are very similar to those experienced when the diagnosis is initially established (Chapter 4). In most instances however, the family, and, in older children, the patient will have to face the harsh reality that the outcome of the disease may well be death. Very often the relative optimism which may have been encouraged by the treating team has now to be converted to pessimism. This is an exceedingly difficult adjustment involving disappointment with the treatment, anger with the disease process and adjustment to the patients inner most feelings about death. The responses of the patient and the family under these circumstances are very variable. There are some guidelines which may prove helpful in this adjustment process.

1. It is essential that the medical implications of the relapse be well understood. This requires an explanation by the medical staff of the relative chances of success of the various treatment options, the likely mode of death with or without treatment, the duration of survival, and the quality of life with or without treatment. A full understanding of this factual information requires more than one discussion with staff.
2. Frequently the various options of management are only slightly different and under the stress of the diagnosis of relapse it may be difficult to make a decision. Under such circumstances, seeking advice from trusted friends or mentors can be very useful.
3. It is necessary to balance the desire to prolong life, or even have a remote chance of cure against the effects of extraordinary treatment methods, on the quality of life. In the case of children who are unable to express their opinion, the family and the treatment team should make every effort to see the treatment options from the child's point of view. In the case of children who can express an opinion, this should be very seriously considered, and no form of treatment should be forced on the child against their expressed will. However, the wish of the child should be taken in the context of the child's maturity, and where all are agreed that a wrong decision has been made by the child, all possible means of persuasion should be employed to correct this decision. Such attempts at persuasion are best made by a person or persons that the child trusts.
4. Unproven and untested methods of treatment euphemistically called "alternative medicine" (see Chapter 5) are at best useless and at worst harmful.

5. Coming to terms with the idea that the illness is incurable cannot happen overnight. Of the many methods of coping with it, one that is most frequently adopted by children of all ages is to live from one day to the next and derive as much satisfaction as possible from each day lived. This is a healthy and useful attitude which should be supported by the family and the professional staff. In this context, treatment methods should be flexible so as to allow the child to enjoy and participate in events which are important to them.
6. Nothing is gained by the "last grand gesture", such as sudden long trips to exotic places. Most children prefer to remain in a familiar environment among their family and friends and close to professional staff who they trust.

CHAPTER 7

Bone Marrow Transplantation

In some situations, the only effective treatment for leukemia or one of the childhood cancers may be the use of near lethal or lethal doses of chemotherapy, or chemotherapy combined with irradiation. These doses are lethal because they permanently destroy the cells of the bone marrow and therefore the patient lacks white blood cells to combat infection and platelets to prevent hemorrhage. To rescue the bone marrow, one of two strategies can be used.

1. Allogeneic transplantation:
   Bone marrow is transplanted from a suitable donor.
2. Autologous transplantation:
   The patients own bone marrow is harvested, frozen and stored in the frozen state before the anti cancer treatment is given and it is returned to the patient after the anti-cancer treatment.

Both methods have certain advantages and disadvantages and these will be discussed later. In effect, bone marrow transplantation is a very sophisticated transfusion.

CHOICE OF DONOR

The individuality of each person is coded in their genetic material and is expressed in the form of an arrangement of complex proteins on cell surfaces which are unique for the individual. These proteins are known as the HLA system and their various subcomponents are known as HLA–A, B, C and D (Figure 14). The presence and exact type of these proteins is detected by antibodies for the A, B and C proteins and by reac-

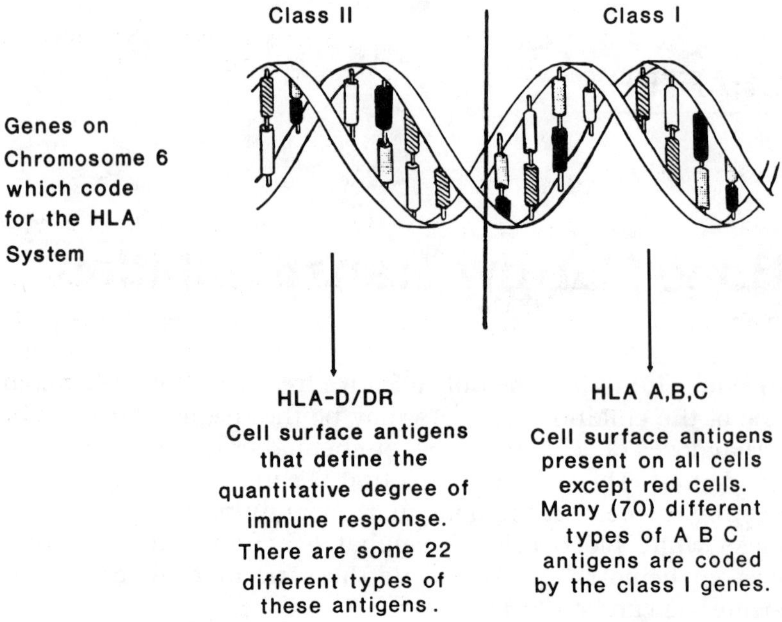

FIGURE 14 HLA System.

tion of lymphocytes against each other (mixed lymphocyte reaction—MLR) for the D proteins. Conceptually, the system is similar to the familiar blood groups A, B, AB and O, but differs from them in that the HLA system is present on all cells and not only red blood cells.

Children inherit their HLA types from the genetic material of each parent as the chromosomes from the spermatozoa and the ovum unite at conception. As a result, except in rare instances, a child has different HLA types from their parents but there is an approximately 1:4 chance that brothers or sisters (siblings) of the child may have the same HLA type. A compatible bone marrow transplant donor is an HLA and MLR matched sibling.

TESTING OF DONORS

Blood is taken from the patient, their siblings and parents, and the HLA types are established in the laboratory. If a HLA–A & B compatible sibling donor is present a second sample of blood is sent to the laboratory to test the identity of the HLA–D locus in the MLR reaction.

Reason for Matched Donors

Rejection of foreign cells occurs by recognition of a foreign HLA arrangement on the cell surface. The massive doses of anti-cancer treatment used in the patient suppresses the patient's immune function, and therefore interfere with rejection of the graft. However, they have no effect on the ability of the grafted lymphocytes to recognize the host as foreign. When an incompatible bone marrow transplant is given, there are two possible consequences.

1. Host rejects graft–graft rejection.
2. Graft rejects host–graft versus host disease (GVHD).

GRAFT VERSUS HOST DISEASE

In situations where a mismatched bone marrow infusion is given to the patient, there follows a severe disease which involves the liver, mouth and gastro-intestinal tract, skin, lungs and a marked increase in susceptibility to infections. The diseases resulting from such a mismatched bone marrow transplant are very distressing and may be fatal. For this reason it is essential that tissue typed matched bone marrow be used for transplantation. Even in tissue matched transplantation, severe forms of GVHD can occur and may be fatal. More often the GVHD is mild and can resolve spontaneously, or be adequately prevented and controlled with the use of drugs such as methotrexate, cyclosporin and prednisone.

In children, GVHD is less common and less severe than in adults. However in mismatched transplants the GVHD is just as severe as in adults. A variety of research techniques is being explored in an effort to widen the scope of bone marrow transplantation from the fully matched sibling, to one with a partial mismatch. So far GVHD or failure of bone marrow engraftment have proven to be major problems with these partially matched transplants.

Anti-leukemic Effect of GVHD

There is good evidence that the frequency of recurrence of acute lymphocytic leukemia after bone transplantation is reduced in the presence of GVHD. Thus GVHD appears to be able to either increase the anti-leukemic effect of the chemotherapy and irradiation, or it exerts a specific anti-leukemic effect of its own.

Types of GVHD

GVHD is classified as *acute* and *chronic*. By definition the acute form of the disease occurs in the first 100 days after transplantation. The chronic form occurs subsequently, with its most severe effects on skin, liver, mouth and a high incidence of serious or even fatal infections. There is a variety of immunosuppressive regimens for its treatment but none are truly effective. In many patients, chronic GVHD is persistent or even fatal, but in about 1/3 it may "burn itself out".

INDICATIONS FOR BONE MARROW TRANSPLANTATION

Acute Lymphocytic Leukemia (ALL): Because bone marrow transplantation is still a young and developing field, hard and fast rules about its use should not be made. Most people agree that it is the treatment of choice when a relapse has occurred during treatment, or within 6 months of stopping treatment. There is also evidence that transplantation in first remission in patients with unfavorable prognostic features (Chapter 10) may increase their chance of cure. There is dispute on the value of transplantation in ALL with more than one relapse, and it is of little value if there have been 2 or more relapses. At present there is no convincing evidence that autologous transplantation is of value in ALL.

Acute Myeloid Leukemia (AML): Both autologous and allogeneic transplantation are of established value in first remission and are widely used. There is at present no convincing evidence which shows that allogeneic transplantation, with its risks of GVHD, is superior to the simpler and safer procedure of autologous transplantation. In AML in relapse, allogeneic transplantation is of value, but autologous transplantation is not.

Chronic Myeloid Leukemia and Myelodysplasias: Allogeneic transplantation is the treatment of choice and whenever possible should be undertaken before these chronic conditions transfer to acute leukemia.

Solid Tumors: The indications for transplantation in the solid tumors of childhood are not yet well defined. Such treatment is only indicated in very advanced tumors (Stage III and IV) and those in which there is some evidence of an increasing sensitivity of the tumor to escalating doses of drugs. At present, autologous bone marrow transplantation appears to be capable of prolonging life or curing some patients with advanced forms of non-Hodgkin's lymphoma, neuroblastoma, Ewing's sarcoma and disseminated retinoblastoma. Allogeneic transplantation has also been used in the treatment of neuroblastoma and Ewing's sarcoma, but appears to have few benefits over autologous transplantation.

PROCEDURE OF TRANSPLANTATION

Informed Consent

The person undergoing transplantation, the donor and their family should have the opportunity of discussing the reasons for transplantation and the risks involved, with a panel of doctors and nurses, or with the doctors of their choice. A decision to embark upon transplantation should not be undertaken in haste. It is important to remember that death from GVHD may be more distressing than death from cancer. The decision-making process in transplantation can be extremely complicated and may require conferences with a wide range of people. It is a great oversimplification to reason that a bone marrow transplant will give a 10% chance of cure and standard therapy only less than 1%, therefore a bone marrow transplant is desirable. Such reasoning fails to take into account the fact that a failed transplant is certain to cause an awful death with no useful quality of life between the procedure of transplantation and death. In decision-making it is necessary to consider not only the chance of survival, but also the quality of remaining life and the quality of death. Where the odds for success of transplantation are poor then a decision for or against transplantation will have to involve, family, social, moral and religious issues. In young children there is the added difficulty that the decision is made for them rather than by them.

Bone Marrow Harvest

This is a relatively simple technique involving multiple bone marrow aspirates undertaken under general anesthesia. The bone marrow is usually obtained from the hip bones only, and the procedure requires an anesthetic for approximately 1–2 hours. Afterwards there is some discomfort in the hip bones but usually this settles within 48 hours. The bone marrow harvest has no harmful effect on the donors bone marrow, with no reduction in the white cell count or platelet counts. Occasionally the volume of marrow aspirated is such that a blood transfusion may be required. Usually however, a blood product such as albumin and oral iron therapy are enough to overcome the blood loss associated with marrow harvest.

Conditioning or Preparative Treatment

This term relates to the choice of anti-cancer drugs which are given immediately before the marrow transplant. The choice of the type of drug and its dose is related to the most effective way of controlling the cancer, as well as suppressing the host's immune system with the least side effects. The choice of such agents is based on experience in a variety of transplantation centers and may differ from one place to another. Two popular regimens that are currently used are fractionated total body irradiation with high dose cyclophosphamide (cytoxan), or high dose Busulphan and Cyclophosphamide without irradiation.

Bone Marrow Infusion

The harvested bone marrow is given to the recipient as a simple intravenous infusion usually through a central venous device e.g. Hickman catheter. The infused cells pass from the circulation into the bone marrow cavity. It is not known why cells settle in the bone marrow cavity in preference to other organs.

After reinfusion, the stem cells of the marrow begin to multiply and differentiate. Recognisable mature cells from the marrow stem cells usually appear in the peripheral blood some 2–3 weeks after transplantation. In patients with allogeneic transplantation, repopulation occurs more rapidly than in those with autologous bone marrow transplantation. This is because in autologous transplantation the harvested marrow has previously been exposed to anti-cancer drugs resulting in a loss of stem cells.

NURSING OF TRANSPLANT PATIENT

Patients undergoing transplantation will require blood products, antibiotics and often intravenous nutrition in the interval between conditioning treatment and recovery of bone marrow function. This can be achieved with least pain and danger by inserting a device which will enable venous access without multiple needling of the veins. Such devices are described in Chapter 4. They are inserted prior to transplantation under a general anesthetic.

Patients undergoing transplantation are in danger of infection. To reduce the risks of infection they are nursed in a protected environment and are handled by staff and relatives who wear gowns and masks and must maintain strict hygiene.

For as long as food can be taken by mouth it is provided in semi-sterile or sterile form (usually canned foods). Dieticians give guidelines on what type of food products are permitted during the phase of toxicity.

Following the conditioning regimen there is a phase of total marrow failure. At this time the patient will require regular transfusions of irradiated blood products e.g. platelets and intravenous broad spectrum antibiotics. The blood products need to be irradiated to prevent the development of GVHD resulting from transfusion of foreign lymphocytes which are present in blood products. It is also desirable to choose as donors of blood products, individuals who are not infected with certain viruses such as cytomegalovirus, Epstein Barr virus, hepatitis or AIDS.

Pain and discomfort often occur during the phase of marrow failure. Mouth ulcers with resultant pain may require a continuous morphine infusion for some days.

In patients with allogeneic transplantation, administration of the drugs which have been chosen to prevent GVHD commences after marrow infusion. Initially they are given intravenously but later by mouth.

Throughout the period of transplantation the patient will require detailed monitoring of blood salts, blood counts, kidney and liver function. If GVHD develops, further complicated tests may be required. The period of intense nursing in an uncomplicated transplant usually lasts for 2 weeks but if complications occur then intensive treatment may continue for 1–6 months.

AFTERCARE

After transplantation, bone marrow function recovers earlier than immune function. As a result there is still a substantial risk of infection despite a normal blood count. In uncomplicated allogeneic transplants normal activities resume in 6 months and in 3–6 months in autologous transplants. The period of isolation from normal activities, contact with members of the peer group, and the many restrictions on diet, free movement and entertainment inevitably take their toll of the child. Emotional maladjustment is common, leading to demanding behavior, altered sleep patterns, sudden bouts of aggression, depression, and rejection of healthy siblings including the donor. These disturbances are usually self limiting and settle once a normal life style can be resumed and the child's appearance returns to normal. When the disturbance is more severe professional help may be required.

SUMMARY

Bone marrow transplantation is a major hazardous procedure for which there are a few absolute and many relative indications. The patient and family embarking on such a program must be aware of its hazards as well as benefits, and be prepared to cope with the prolonged periods of sickness and limitations of normal activity. In allogeneic transplantation there is a serious risk of GVHD. Transplantation cannot guarantee a cure of the disease, but in some instances it gives the patient their best chance of cure.

CHAPTER 8

Unproven and Untested Methods of Treatment

These masquerade under many titles, including "alternative medicine", and are practised by a variety of people some with training, and others without any formal health science education. They have no system of registration, or professional quality control, and no national or international system of information exchange based on scientific method and strict peer review. Some of its practitioners are genuinely, even fiercely, convinced of the truth and importance of their methods of treatment, while others are charlatans.

RESULTS OF TREATMENT

Practitioners of that form of treatment almost always tell anecdotes of unexpected cures achieved with their method of treatment. What they never do is to provide well documented comparisons of methods of treatment, or a strict assessment of the stage and microscopic type of the disease in their patients, who they claim have been successfully treated. They also have no plausible rationale for their treatment method beyond vague statements on the major effects of diet, stress and immunity. When these notions are examined for good evidence of scientific proof they are found to be nothing more than hypotheses, or poorly understood failed scientific postulates. The reports of their treatment methods are unpublished in scientific journals, and claims are made that there is a conspiracy to suppress their publication because they contradict the value of proven methods of treatment.

A variety of national and international panels have examined the claims of cure by these practitioners. These include committees consisting of lay, medical, scientific and government representatives. Their universal assessment is that the number of cures does not exceed that expected to be seen by chance alone. In the experience of the author and his colleagues no child or adult receiving treatment from these people has achieved a cure or even an unexpected prolonged remission.

ROLE OF "ALTERNATIVE TREATMENT"

Alternative treatments have always been offered and have been accepted in some patients with cancer. This indicates that in these people they cater for certain deep seated irrational hopes, such as miracle cures. People who desire to seek additional treatment for their child with cancer from such sources will probably not be satisfied until they have tried them. It is however important for their child's sake to remember certain principles which ensure that the child's best interests remain foremost.

1. If the child is old enough they should be consulted on whether or not they wish to see yet another "health practitioner".
2. Scientific medical treatment should not be stopped, postponed or altered, and the treatment advocated by the "alternative" practitioner should not counteract the effects of scientific medical treatment.
3. The "alternative" treatment should not turn the child with cancer into a "cancer child". Life should not be lived with the thought of disease and fear of death all the time.
4. The family should beware of major financial commitment such as that entailed in travel and lodgment in places owned or managed by the "alternative" practitioners, and the purchase of expensive diets and medications available only from their sources.
5. Arrangements should be made with reputable health agencies or doctors to provide for terminal care so that the child is not deprived of pain control and appropriate nursing

facilities when the treatment has failed and death is inevitable.

TYPES OF "ALTERNATIVE TREATMENTS"

There is a wide range of such treatments. The most common are dietary regimens and herbal treatments. Less often certain "alternative treatment" practitioners claim to have discovered a universal cure for cancer based on their discovery of the miraculous properties of a vitamin or chemical (e.g. Vitamin C, Lactrile, retinoic acid), or a type of medical treatment that had been popularized by the press (e.g. immunotherapy). At the other end of the spectrum are alternative practitioners who use their personality and religious beliefs to attempt faith healing, or healing through meditation.

In general dietary regimens, herbal treatments and meditation are least harmful to children. Most harmful are the peddlers of miracle cures because they raise false hopes and when these are shattered they transfer the responsibility of failure onto the patient and the family. This is done by implying that the treatment failed because it was sought too late or that there was failure to comply with all the details of treatment.

CHAPTER 9

The Dying Child

Unfortunately, in some children all attempts at cure fail, and after a protracted illness death becomes inevitable. In other circumstances the malignancy presents with overwhelming disease which is fatal before effective anti-cancer treatment can be commenced. Under still other circumstances, unexpected death occurs during the course of treatment as a result of a complication of the malignancy or its treatment. The preparation of the child and the family for impending death, coping with the process of death and its aftermath is heavily dependent on the social, ethnic, religious, ethical and psychological status of the individuals concerned. It is not possible or desirable to try to produce a set of universal guidelines which can be applied to all circumstances related to death. What follows is the authors point of view, based on his personal background and experience with children and families confronting death.

For convenience, and because of real differences in reactions and coping mechanisms, it is best to subdivide this subject into:

1. death after a protracted illness;
2. death at the beginning of the illness;
3. unexpected death during the treatment of malignancy.

DEATH AFTER A PROTRACTED ILLNESS

As has already been discussed in Chapter 6, relapse of the cancer usually signifies to the family that death is inevitable.

As with the initial diagnosis of cancer or with relapse there may be phases of rejection, depression, transient euphoria and a search for miracle cures, but in the majority of families, in a matter of weeks or months a transformation occurs with acceptance of the inevitability of death. In some instances, the pursuit of a variety of alternative medical treatments may become an obsession, and may lead to unnecessary additional hardships for the family and the patient. It is necessary under these difficult circumstances to point out to the family the obsessive and counterproductive nature of their efforts, in the hope that with time they will be able to accept the reality and take appropriate steps to prepare the child and themselves for the child's death.

PREPARING FOR DEATH

It is at this stage that the crucial decision to share the burdens of the terminal illness must be made. One should be prepared to mobilize and use all the resources of the family, the local community, and the treatment center. Withdrawal by the family into a very private grief only aggravates the stresses placed on the patient and the family, and retards the healing process. Fortunately, attitudes to death in cancer among the community and professionals have changed as a result of the writings and teaching of a number of concerned and dedicated pioneers in this field, and with this change there have developed a number of community based self-help groups. These groups usually maintain contact with the treatment center and can be contacted by the medical social worker attached to the treatment center. A variety of organizations affiliated with religious denominations also often exist in the local community, and can be very helpful in arranging help for meals at home, baby sitting and transport. Community nurses and family doctors may provide practical advice on coping with the many symptoms of the terminal illness such as pain control, constipation, nausea and vomiting, and altered sleep habits.

The extended family can also be of great assistance during the terminal phase. Overall, it is best to arrange a series of practical tasks for the extended family and rely on professionals for psychological support.

APPROACH TO THE DYING CHILD

When a number of attempts at curative treatment have failed, the child gradually realizes that they will not be cured. When this happens there is initially resignation to frequent bouts of poor health. Subsequently, the child becomes tired of the poor quality of life that they are leading and often seem to long for death. The child's passage through these phases can be assisted by an honest discussion of the failed treatment regimens, and why other ones are unlikely to be successful. Attention is focussed on quality of life issues. This is done by using medications in such a way as to allow the child to participate in pleasant events, and by effective treatment of symptoms such as pain, constipation and sleeplessness.

CONTROL OF SYMPTOMS

Unfortunately, with time the symptoms of the disease become disabling to such an extent that normal activities can no longer be undertaken, and the child's waking hours are dominated by the disease. This is a very distressing phase of the terminal illness and one which requires a good deal of attention from doctors and nurses in order to treat the symptoms. Most important is control of pain. The mainstay of pain control is morphine or one of its derivatives given in a regular schedule with gradually increasing doses. In addition to morphine, control of pain can be improved by the use of aspirin and non-steroidal anti-inflammatory agents. For these drugs to be most effective they should be administered on a regular 4–6 hourly schedule rather than only when the pain is severe.

The use of morphine or its derivatives on a long term basis is associated with a change of sleeping habits. The normal sleep rhythm is reversed, with the patient being drowsy during the day and awake at night. The use of hypnotics to assist return to normal sleep pattern is usually unsuccessful. It is better to make arrangements to keep the child amused and occupied during the night hours rather than to force them to sleep.

A side effect of the morphine group of drugs is constipation. This can be a distressing additional symptom of the terminal illness. The use of laxatives and occasional enemas can relieve this complications.

There are also aberration of appetite. In most children there is a loss of interest in food and drink. Nothing is gained by trying to cajole the child to eat. In most children there are sudden desires for unusual foods. Whenever possible these should be indulged, even though in most instances only a few mouthfuls are eaten.

EMOTIONAL NEEDS

The major need of terminally ill children is to be not lonely, and to be in an environment which is familiar to them and in which they feel safe. Almost always such an environment can be best achieved in the child's home. To create the appropriate environment it is best for both parents to be at home as much as possible, and to station the child in the center of the home close to all other members of the family within the living area. When the child desires peace and quiet they can temporarily be moved to a bedroom. Occasionally the symptoms of the illness become very distressing and cannot be controlled at home despite the intervention of professional help. Under such circumstances a temporary short time admission to the treatment center is desirable in order to stabilize the child on a new dose of morphine, or to institute other palliative measures. Such short admissions to a familiar treatment center are welcomed by the child. On the other hand, admissions for palliative care into unfamiliar surroundings are very frightening to the child and seldom achieve the desired result. In some countries hospices have been established for children. They appear to play a role in certain circumstances by functioning as a "home away from home". The key issue is to ensure that the child is in the bosom of the family and is never lonely.

All members of the family should be encouraged to participate in the terminal care of the child. This is particularly important for the child's brothers and sisters. No matter what age, they should be given the opportunity to perform some tasks to help the dying child. It must also be appreciated that sibling rivalry and arguments may persist during the terminal illness, and that some gentle intervention by the parents may be required when the dying child becomes irritable or overtired because of the behavior of the siblings.

A terminally ill child becomes resigned to death and is seldom afraid of it. The siblings on the other hand frequently have no idea of death. It is wise to discuss the process of death with the siblings and compare it to falling into a permanent sleep, introducing whatever religious modifications are considered desirable by the family.

Some teenagers and adolescents express the desire to talk about death and to arrange for the distribution of their possessions after death. They should be encouraged to do so with the person or persons with whom they have formed the best relationship. Under no circumstances should they be lied to by denying that they are dying. Conversations about death should be left to their initiative and should range only as widely as desired by the patient.

Expression of emotion during the terminal process is healthy. Initiation of expression of emotion should be in the hands of the patient. If they wish to weep, then someone should assist them and weep with them. If they wish to be angry, their anger should be heard in silence and without argument or denial.

THE MOMENT OF DEATH

Contrary to popular belief the moment of death is not dramatic. It really is akin to falling asleep. There is often a preceding phase of semi-consciousness with brief waking moments and then a change of breathing with intermittent deep breaths, which become less frequent and finally cease. It is at this stage that the heart beat ceases and the person is no longer rousable. Witnessing the process is not frightening and can be very well accepted by adults and children.

CONFIRMATION OF DEATH

This is undertaken by a medical officer and is required by the legal authorities in virtually all countries. The treatment center often makes arrangements with the local medical officer for the signature of the death certificate.

FUNERAL ARRANGEMENTS

In most instances arrangements would have been made with undertakers for the funeral. In most societies these arrangements can be simply made by a telephone call to the undertakers who will collect the child's body from home after the appropriate certification of death. If a child dies in hospital the procedure is very similar, with the child's body being first placed in the hospital mortuary and then taken by the undertakers to the funeral parlor.

AUTOPSY

In many instances the doctors will ask the family for permission for autopsy. Autopsy can more accurately determine the cause of death than any of the investigations which were undertaken during life. The results of autopsy can also advance some aspects of medical science. The decision to permit or refuse autopsy is finally determined by the family.

FUNERAL

At the time of death it is desirable for all members of the family and particularly the siblings to view the child's body. The siblings also participate in the funeral. Open expression of grief should be encouraged, and questions posed by the siblings about the disease and death answered.

DELAYED REACTIONS TO DEATH

The parents of a child who died after a prolonged illness have been under a great deal of stress during the illness and the dying process. A variety of reactions to this stress occurs but are often restricted by pressure of circumstances. After death the immediacy of the situation diminishes, and the stresses and strains which developed during the course of the illness can surface. This can prove to be a very difficult time for the parents because of feelings of guilt, recrimination and anger. Attitudes toward work, friends and the local community may undergo dramatic and fluctuating changes. Personal relationships between husband and wife may alter greatly. The degree to which these problems dominate the life's of the family differ from one family to another, and to some extent their severity depends on pre-existing stresses in the family.

There are no easy answers to these problems. When they are mild and the reasons for them are understood by both parents they usually resolve with time. Where the tensions are severe and there are signs of a breakup of the family, then it is imperative to arrange for counselling with a trained grief or crisis counsellor. In many instances such counselling can, over a period of time, help the whole family to recover from the consequences of the fatal illness. Arrangements for appropriate counselling can often be made through members of the cancer treatment team.

DEATH AT THE ONSET OF THE ILLNESS

The major difference here is that the parents and siblings of the child have had no time to prepare themselves for the patient's death. The patient is usually not aware of being terminally ill and most often dies in an unconscious state. It is the family that most acutely suffer the consequences of death. Unfortunately in many circumstances, such a family is totally unprepared for the death of the child, and are unable to mobilize the resources of help that exist in the community and treatment centers. This process must be undertaken by health professionals and is best handled by professional grief or crisis counsellors. Families that lose their children at the beginning of an illness have more in common with families who lose children through accidents, than through a prolonged illness and should be directed to appropriate self help groups in their community.

UNEXPECTED DEATH DURING TREATMENT

This is always a devastating situation for the family and for the treatment team. Such children usually develop a sudden severe illness for which they are given every available medical treatment but die without having the opportunity to realize that they are dying. The family is initially bewildered but hopeful that recovery will take place. It is confronted by an overwhelming array of "high tech" equipment and specialists trying to cope with the next devastating complication. In the circumstances there may be very little time to mobilize family and community resources. It is possible to alleviate some of these problems by ensuring that the parents maintain close contact with a doctor of the cancer treatment team who has a good appreciation of the likely outcome of the illness, and can warn the parents as soon as possible the likelihood of death.

As with death at home, it is desirable that all the family and the siblings have an opportunity to see the fatally ill child either before or, as soon as feasible, after death.

In most instances an autopsy is highly desirable, not only to advance medical science but also to answer the very important question—namely, why did this catastrophe happen? The best way to answer this question is to reconstruct, in the light of the autopsy findings, the circumstances that have led to death.

Unexpected death during the course of the illness arouses two difficult emotional responses which usually do not occur under the other circumstances.

1. Anger

   It is perfectly natural for the parents and the family to feel anger and to wish to channel it in some direction. It is better to express this anger openly to the appropriate persons, than to suppress or internalize it. It is wise to wait for a full factual explanation of the circumstances causing death before taking recriminatory actions.

2. Guilt

   Self criticism by the treatment team is also a very understandable and desirable feeling after an unexpected death. Review of the circumstances leading to such a death may help prevent it occurring again.

Specific Conditions

CHAPTER 10

Acute Lymphocytic Leukemia—ALL

This is the most common of the childhood malignancies. Dramatic improvements in methods of treatment have transformed this condition from one which was almost always fatal, to one which can be cured in the majority of children.

DIAGNOSIS

The doctors suspect the diagnosis on the basis of the medical history. There is often pallor, tiredness and irritability. Bruising may be prominent but bleeding is rare. When the child is examined, the doctors look for enlargement of the spleen, liver and lymph nodes. A blood examination very often gives the diagnosis, but it must be confirmed by a bone marrow aspirate. This is the only way to obtain a sufficient number of truly primitive cells which can be studied for likely response to treatment and give clues to the likely long term outlook.

The bone marrow aspirate shows virtually complete replacement of normal bone marrow cells by primitive cells which are called leukemia blasts. A close inspection of these leukemic blasts shows identifying features which allow classification of the cells into one of 3 types which have been called by a French-American-British team of experts as L1, L2 and L3. This is called the FAB classification. A high proportion of L1 cells is often associated with a good response to treatment. More than 10–25% of L2 cells is generally considered as indicating that intense treatment is required. Cells with L3 features are associated with a type of leukemia known as "B" cell leukemia which is often associated with genetic changes suggestive of a poor prognosis with standard treatment.

STAGING

Leukemia is always a widespread disease. It is however, necessary to know whether there is infiltration of the central nervous system. This can be determined with the first spinal tap. In addition, in some circumstances there may be a suspicion that the glands inside the chest cavity or the kidneys have been infiltrated. Under these circumstances a chest x-ray and/or abdominal ultrasound examination are urgent investigations.

PROGNOSTIC FACTORS

If there are unfavorable prognostic features treatment can be altered in an attempt to improve the outlook. Table 3 gives an indication of the more important established prognostic features.

Other very important poor prognostic features are the presence of leukemic cell involvement of the central nervous system, or the failure to respond to chemotherapy.

Prognostic features only indicate *probabilities* and they can change when new and better treatment methods are developed. The more effective the treatment of the disease, the less significant are the prognostic features.

OUTLINE OF TREATMENT

Most treatment centers follow a well defined and carefully structured and tested protocol. Adherence to these protocols has been one of the main reasons for the current success of treatment. The mainstay of treatment is *chemotherapy*. The general principle is that the early treatment must be intensive using at least 3–4 chemotherapeutic agents with other ones introduced later. Early treatment of the central nervous system with chemotherapy administered by spinal taps is essential. Some form of treatment of leukemia for the brain is required in most but not all children. This may consist of irradiation or chemotherapy given in an intensive manner. Some form of con-

TABLE 3

Prognostic features in ALL.

Factor	*Favorable*	*Unfavorable*
Age < 1 year		+++
Age > 10 years		+
Age 2–9 years	++	
White cell count > 100,000		+++
White cell count < 10,000	++	
FAB classification		
L1	++	
L2		++
L3		+++
"B" cell leukemia		+++
"T" cell leukemia		+
"Common ALL antigen positive"	++	
Hyperdiploid (more than 50 chromosomes)	+++	
Translocation of chromosomes		+++

tinuation treatment which is less intensive than the early treatment is required, most probably for no longer than 2 years.

The treatment is usually broken down into phases.

Phase I – *remission induction* usually lasts 4–6 weeks.

Phase II – *central nervous system therapy* usually lasts 4–6 weeks.

Phase III – *consolidation* or reinduction and reconsolidation. Lasts for variable time intervals depending on the type of treatment protocol.

Phase IV – *continuation therapy*—usually lasts for 2 years.

Each treatment center will have its own definitions and time intervals for the above phases of treatment. All major treatment centers have written protocols which have been determined by groups of doctors, scientists and statisticians. These protocols ensure that the most up to date information is used for the benefit of the patient. Since there is no single method of treatment which cures all children with leukemia, the protocols are often designed to ask questions related to treatment. Such protocols usually involve a randomized study. This means that the selection of one or other type of treatment is done on the basis of chance alone. It is worth repeating that the types of treatment which are under investigation are only incorporated into a protocol if it is certain that they will not harm the child.

The following is a list of drug names which are often used in the various phases of treatment:

Phase I	Vincristine	
	Prednisone	
	Anthracyclines—	Daunomycin
		Adriamycin
	Asparaginase	
	Spinal taps using methotrexate.	
Phase II	Spinal taps with methotrexate	
	Cranial irradiation or intravenous methotrexate	
	Cyclophosphamide (Cytoxan)	
	Vincristine	
	6 mercaptopurine	
	Cytosine Arabinoside (Ara–C).	
Phase III	High dose asparaginase or modified regimens similar to phase I and II	
	Various other intermediate or high dose single agents e.g. methotrexate or Ara–C.	
Phase IV	Usually oral drugs e.g. 6 mercaptopurine and methotrexate with boosters of vincristine and prednisone.	

COMPLICATIONS

These can be of two main types:

1. those of the disease and

2. those of treatment.

It is most convenient to think of these according to the phase of treatment.

Phase I – The leukemia has suppressed normal bone marrow function as a result of which the child is susceptible to infection and hemorrhage. They may also be anemic. In most children transfusion of platelets and red cells will be required, and in 75% it will be necessary to use intravenous antibiotics. Occasionally the side effects of the chemotherapy may become a problem. The most significant ones, and the drugs which are mainly responsible are listed according to the phase of treatment below:

Drug	**Side Effect**
Vincristine	Abdominal pain and constipation
	Weakness and tingling of legs
Prednisone	Rapid weight gain
	Changes in mood
	Diabetes
Asparaginase	Allergy
	Diabetes
	Disturbance of blood clotting
	Abdominal pain due to inflammation of pancreas.
Anthracyclines	Nausea and vomiting
	Mouth ulcers
	Difficulty with swallowing.

Note that hair loss is most commonly due to vincristine and anthracyclines.

Phase II – The main side effects of drugs most often used in this phase are shown below.

Cyclophosphamide (Cytoxan)	Nausea and vomiting Blood in urine.
Cytosine Arabinoside (Ara–C)	Nausea and vomiting Mouth ulcers.

Radiation	Headache "Somnolence syndrome" i.e. drowsiness, loss of appetite and depression lasting 1–2 weeks some 6–8 weeks after treatment when irradiation is completed.

Phase III – At this time the child is usually well, with a normally functioning bone marrow. The side effects now relate to using particularly high doses of drugs to ensure maximum cell kill.

Drug	**Side Effect**
High dose methotrexate (often also used in Phase II)	Mouth ulcers Loss of appetite Liver damage Skin Rash
High dose Asparaginase	Allergy Abdominal pain Diabetes Loss of appetite and depression
High dose Cytosine Arabinoside (Ara–c)	Conjunctivitis Mouth ulcers Nausea and vomiting Difficulty with balance.

Phase IV – There is seldom much drug related toxicity during this phase. Occasionally 6 mercaptopurine or methotrexate may be associated with impaired liver function, or there may be a need to reduce doses because of persistent suppression of bone marrow function.

CESSATION OF TREATMENT

There is good evidence that continuing treatment for longer than 2 years does not decrease the risk of leukemia recurrence. Before treatment is stopped it is necessary to perform a bone marrow aspirate and spinal tap to ensure that the patient is in remission.

"When is a Child with Leukemia Cured?"

Leukemia can recur after treatment is stopped even if the bone marrow and spinal taps show no leukemic cells. This is because the above tests are only a representative picture of the state of the whole bone marrow or the central nervous system. When there are only small numbers of residual leukemia cells in the bone marrow or central nervous system, the chance of them being discovered by a bone marrow aspirate or spinal tap is remote.

Recurrence of leukemia occurs mainly in the first two years after cessation of treatment. At present the recurrence rate is 15–20% with 99.9% of the recurrences occurring within 2 years of stopping treatment.

For practical purposes therefore the chance of recurrence of leukemia is 0.1% or less two years after treatment has stopped. This is such a low figure that it is reasonable to assume that the child has been cured. Strictly speaking cure could be defined as a risk of recurrence of leukemia which is no greater than the incidence of leukemia in the general population. If this definition is used, cure cannot be claimed until 4 years from cessation of treatment.

Another and possibly more important concept of cure is the "true cure". True cure implies not only no recurrence of the disease but also a return to the same state of physical and psychological health that may have existed had the disease never occurred. While this is desirable, it is probably not achievable.

LONG TERM COMPLICATIONS OF TREATMENT

It is still too early to be sure that all the long term complications of treatment of leukemia have been reported. In general it must be stressed that long term complications are surprisingly rare.

Physical Complications

Their presence or absence is largely determined by whether or not irradiation to the cranium and/or spine were part of the treatment protocol, the dose of irradiation, and the child's age at the time of irradiation. Those children who received irradiation to the skull tend to have a somewhat reduced circumference of the head and slightly, or moderately, reduced final body height. There is a tendency to an excessive appetite leading to obesity. These symptoms are most apparent with higher doses of irradiation (2400 rad or 24Gy), and in children who were younger than 9 years when irradiated.

In those who received irradiation of the cranium and spine there is always a reduction of height with a relatively short spine compared with the length of the arms and legs. In addition there are also the symptoms outlined above for children who received cranial irradiation only.

Apart from the above physical problems there are remarkably few other side effects. In some children scalp hair is sparse, particularly if they required more than one course of irradiation, or if they received irradiation and a class of anti-leukemic drugs known as the anthracyclines. Fertility remains normal in girls and boys, and there is no evidence that their children suffer from an increased rate of congenital malformations.

So far, second cancers have been reported in a small number of children and these have been mainly certain types of brain tumors. They have only been reported in children who received irradiation of the skull.

Psychological Complications

These are again most common in those children who received irradiation and spinal taps as part of their treatment. They are most severe in those who were younger than 3 years at the time of irradiation. The disturbance involves a reduced concentration span and short term memory. This in turn makes it difficult for the child to cope with subjects that require a good deal of concentration and memorizing. In practice, the major difficulties are seen in mathematics and the sciences. The disability becomes more marked with time, and is only apparent in later school years. This complication is due to organic brain damage. It cannot be overcome by extra tuition in the "weak" subjects. In fact, extra efforts in these "weak" subjects remain largely unrewarded, and lead to disillusionment by the child with education as a whole. It is therefore far better to accept these learning difficulties and to concentrate efforts on the child's "strong" subjects. This approach leads to a happier school life and better long term accommodation into society. A good deal of assistance in reaching these educational adjustments can be obtained from educational psychologists and experienced teachers once they understand the organic nature of this disability.

There are, of course, many other psychological long term complications, but it is remarkable how rare they are. In general, children cured of leukemia are normal well adjusted young people, with a healthy attitude to life. As adolescents, they often face the problem that their parents are unduly concerned about their well being and safety. In general the difficulties of adolescence have been less marked than in their siblings, perhaps because these children are emotionally more mature than their chronological age.

RELAPSE

Recurrence of leukemia (relapse) is the most serious complication confronting the patient and the family. Relapse can be classified according to the site, and time after treatment at which it occurred.

On the basis of site there are three types:

1. Medullary—those only in the bone marrow.
2. Extramedullary—those only outside the bone marrow, e.g. CNS, testes, iris.
3. Those which are medullary and extramedullary.

On the basis of time they can be divided into 2 types:

1. Those occurring during treatment or within 6 months of ceasing treatment.
2. Those occurring more than 6 months after ceasing treatment.

In general it can be said that extramedullary relapses have a good chance of total cure, and that the longer after cessation of treatment any type of relapse occurs, the better the chance of cure.

Extramedullary Relapse more than 6 Months after Ceasing Treatment

These occur most often in the CNS, testes, eye, or peripheral nerves. The chance of cure is better than 80%. The treatment involves irradiation to the involved site, a series of spinal taps if the involved site is the CNS, and a course of chemotherapy. The precise nature of chemotherapy and its duration depend on the individual treatment unit, and vary from 6 months to 2 years.

Extramedullary Relapse during Treatment or within 6 Months of Ceasing Treatment

Provided that bone marrow aspirate excludes bone marrow relapse, the prognosis for cure remains nearly 80% and the approach to treatment is the same as outlined above. There is, however, an increased risk of medullary relapse, particularly in the first 6 months.

Medullary Relapse more than 6 Months after Ceasing Treatment

The prognosis is much worse than with an extramedullary relapse. In general, 30–40% of children can achieve a cure. This can be accomplished with a repeat course of intensive chemotherapy and spinal taps or by undertaking bone marrow transplantation if a suitable donor is available. The advantages of bone marrow transplantation are that the treatment is completed more quickly but its disadvantages are the risk of GVHD or death from the procedure (see Chapter 7). In most instances a repeat course of chemotherapy is the preferred option.

Medullary Relapse during Treatment or within 6 Months of Ceasing Treatment

This is the most serious of all situations. The prognosis with a change of chemotherapy is very poor with only very rare cures. In this situation there is no doubt that bone marrow transplantation offers the best chance of cure. The chance of cure with a transplant is in the vicinity of 30–40% and the later the relapse has occurred the better the chance of cure.

Medullary and Extramedullary Relapse

The prognosis is as with medullary relapse. Transplantation provides the best chance of cure. If transplantation is possible, then the irradiation program for the extramedullary relapse must be carefully planned so that the organ involved in the relapse does not receive excessive doses of irradiation. If the medullary and extramedullary relapse occur more than 6 months after cessation of treatment, a repeat course of chemotherapy and irradiation to the organ involved in the relapse may achieve a 30–40% chance of cure.

CHAPTER 11

Acute Non-lymphocytic Leukemia (ANL) or Acute Myeloblastic Leukemia (AML)

This is a less common type of leukemia in childhood making up some 15–20% of all the leukemias. Major advances in treatment have made this previously incurable condition now curable in at least 50% of children.

DIAGNOSIS

The diagnosis is suspected on a medical history of bleeding, bruising and pallor. Examination may reveal enlarged liver, spleen and lymph nodes and occasionally the presence of lumps of tumor in other organs including the gums. A blood and bone marrow examination are essential to confirm the suspicion and to permit accurate monitoring of the progress of treatment.

STAGING

As with ALL it is necessary to determine whether there is infiltration of the central nervous system by means of a spinal tap. The bone marrow is processed to determine the structure of the chromosomes, because the various type of ANLL have characteristic chromosome changes. When the patient is treated, the disappearance of these chromosome changes is a sensitive indicator that a remission has been achieved. As with ALL these leukemias are classified into various FAB sub-types but, these do not have prognostic significance.

PROGNOSTIC FACTORS

The clinical and laboratory features are not as good a guide to response to treatment as they are in ALL. With modern treatment methods (see below), only age under 1 year, the presence of CNS involvement at diagnosis and the presence of a chromosome abnormality known as the Philadelphia Chromosome are bad prognostic features.

OUTLINE OF TREATMENT

From the beginning the treatment is very intensive, and is aimed at profound marrow suppression so as to permanently eradicate the leukemia cells. Not only are multiple drugs in high doses required, but in addition they must be given as frequently as is compatible with the patients' survival. This means that the patient must remain in hospital for a prolonged period of time, frequently for as long as 4 weeks. During this time it is almost certain that antibiotics and blood products will be required.

The details of treatment and the choice of drugs will vary from one specialized unit to the next. As with ALL, the treatment centers will have established protocols which will be followed, and which are structured to achieve the maximum possible success. Most of these protocols use combinations of drugs which include moderate or high doses of cytosine arabinoside and one or both anthracyclines. The side effects of these drugs have already been discussed in the previous chapter.

TRANSPLANTATION

There is general agreement that the best results in this type of leukemia are achieved when intensive, potentially lethal antileukemia therapy is used after remission has been achieved. In order to rescue the patient from this type of radical treatment, some form of marrow transplantation is required. Details of transplantation are discussed in Chapter 7.

With intensive chemotherapy induction programs, and either allogeneic or autologous bone marrow transplantation, cure from leukemia can be achieved in at least 50% of patients. The proportion of cures is even higher and may be in the range of

80–100% in those patients who have achieved a stable remission and received allogeneic or autologous bone marrow transplantation. Thus a disease which only a few years ago was regarded as incurable is now curable in at least half the patients, although, only after very intensive treatment. It remains incurable only when compromises and easy options are used in treatment e.g. low drug doses to avoid toxicity or prolonged intervals between chemotherapy for patient or hospital convenience.

COMPLICATIONS OF TREATMENT

These may result from the disease or its treatment. They are best considered according to the phase of treatment.

Induction Therapy

In patients with very high white cell counts there is a risk of brain hemorrhage and blockage of the kidneys from the breakdown products of the cell. A variety of measures may be used to lower these risks. It is always necessary to insert an intravenous drip and give high doses of fluids together with agents that prevent kidney damage. To lower the white cell count it may be necessary to do a form of exchange transfusion. In some patients with certain types of ANL there may be a severe bleeding tendency which will require treatment with certain types of concentrated blood products as well as platelet transfusions. While these measures are usually successful, children with white cell counts in excess of 500,000 have a significant early mortality from brain hemorrhage.

Infection is also frequently present at the time of presentation and requires vigorous antibiotic treatment. Sometimes white cell transfusions may be required in addition to antibiotics to control infection.

Treatment with anti-leukemic drugs is certain to temporarily wipe out any remaining normal bone marrow cells for a period of 2–3 weeks during which time the patient is particularly susceptible to infection. This is the phase of dependence on intensive treatment such as frequent platelet transfusions and a variety of intravenous antibiotics. In children with a poor nutritional status, intravenous feeding may be required.

In addition to the above almost universal complications, some patients also have special drug related toxicity. The most common is mouth ulceration, and this may be accompanied by difficulty and pain on swallowing. This complication is usually caused by the anthracycline drugs (daunomycin, adriamycin) or less often by cytosine arabinoside. If ulceration extends to the whole gastro-intestinal system, there may be diarrhoea and abdominal pain and this may lead to difficult diagnostic problems. Consultation with surgeons may be necessary when there is a possibility of perforation of the oesophagus or the bowel.

The induction phase is fraught with a variety of major medical problems and can only be satisfactorily managed in large specialized departments with experience and access to appropriate personnel and technical equipment.

Consolidation

The phase of induction often lasts 4 weeks during which time the patient achieves remission and with it bone marrow function returns to normal. In the consolidation phase, toxicity is mainly related to the choice of drugs. Most often the toxicity is to the bone marrow causing a tendency to infection and bleeding which is less severe than during the induction phase.

Transplantation

This is discussed in detail in the chapter 7. While it is a very toxic aspect of treatment it is often less frightening to the child and the family because they have become familiar with the toxic effects of treatment. Nevertheless all the resources of the patient and the family will need to be mobilized to cope with the major demands of an uncertain outcome, prolonged isolation nursing, minor unforeseen complications and occasionally major complications of transplantation.

CONTINUATION THERAPY

In some centers it is considered that intensive continuation chemotherapy is as effective as transplantation. These centers use multiple intensive courses of drug combinations. The side effects from this type of treatment are similar to those during consolidation therapy. Continuation therapy is not used after bone marrow transplantation because it is too toxic and is unlikely to have significant benefit.

CESSATION OF TREATMENT

This occurs after bone marrow transplantation. The time for induction, consolidation and bone marrow transplantation varies from one center to another, but the usual range is 6–9 months. If continuation therapy is employed it is usual to stop treatment after 12 months.

CURE

As with ALL there are various definitions of cure. The great majority of relapses occur within 1–2 years of ceasing treatment. In patients with allogeneic bone marrow transplantation, the incidence of relapse is less than 20%, and virtually all occur within 1 year of transplantation. In patients with autologous transplantation the figure for relapse is less reliable, but ranges from 0–50%. The more recent data suggest that the relapse rate is no higher than with allogeneic transplantation i.e. less than 20%. In patients treated with continuation therapy relapses may occur for 2 years after cessation of treatment. Thus, as with ALL, the risks of relapse beyond 2 years after discontinuing treatment are so small as to make it reasonable to consider the patient cured.

LONG TERM COMPLICATIONS

Physical

These are almost entirely related to the modality of treatment used in the conditioning regimen for transplantation. If total body irradiation was used, then there will usually be retardation of growth, sterility and cataracts. The incidence of second tumors is unknown because there have been insufficient numbers of patients followed up for more than 10 years. Patients not treated with irradiation have so far been remarkably free of any long term side effects but as with irradiation, the numbers followed for more than 10 years are very small.

Psychological

Unlike ALL there are no learning difficulties unless the brain required irradiation in excess of that delivered in preparation for transplantation. Other emotional problems are the same as described in the chapter 10 and are usually minor.

RELAPSE

In ANLL some 10–20% of children fail to come into remission and another 10% have a very short lasting remission called an unstable remission. Their chance of cure is virtually nil unless they can be transplanted from an allogeneic donor. In those who can be so transplanted, the chance of cure is approximately 20%. In patients who relapsed when treated with chemotherapy only, the chance of cure with subsequent allogeneic transplantation is 40–50%. In patients who relapse after allogeneic transplantation there is virtually no chance of cure by another transplant. In patients who relapsed after autologous transplantation, there should be a chance of cure with allogeneic transplantation, but there are insufficient numbers of such patients to make any numerical statements.

Extramedullary Relapses

These are far less common in ANL than ALL and if they occur they do so most often in a sub-type of ANL known as acute monocytic leukemia (FAB type M5). The treatment is with local irradiation and chemotherapy for a period of 6–12 months.

CHAPTER 12

Chronic Myeloid Leukemia, Juvenile Chronic Myeloid Leukemia and Myelodysplasia

These are malignant disorders of the most primitive bone marrow stem cells. In most cases of chronic myeloid leukemia there is a characteristic chromosome abnormality known as the Philadelphia chromosome. Juvenile chronic myeloid leukemia and the myelodysplasias are really one and the same disorder in childhood. Some children with these disorders have characteristic chromosome abnormalities, but in others such abnormalities have not yet been defined. In general these disorders are extremely resistant to conventional treatment with chemotherapy, but can be cured in a high proportion of patients by allogeneic transplantation.

CHRONIC MYELOID LEUKEMIA

This usually presents in older boys and girls, and is first noticed because of an increasing abdominal girth which is due to a very large spleen. A blood examination reveals a very high white cell count with the majority of cells having a normal mature appearance. There is no anemia or bleeding tendency. A bone marrow aspirate shows a gross preponderance of white over red cells. In the bone marrow the Philadelphia chromosome can be identified by special cytogenetic techniques. This chromosome is a translocation involving chromosome 9 and 22, abbreviated to t9;22.

TREATMENT

Initial treatment is required to lower the white cell count and reduce the size of the spleen. This can usually be achieved by using a mild chemotherapy regimen given in the form of tablets. Occasionally the spleen fails to shrink adequately, and in these patients other treatment measures such as irradiation or surgical removal may be required.

With this approach to treatment the average survival is 3 years because eventually there is a metamorphosis from the chronic to an acute leukemia which is rapidly fatal. The only way of preventing these complications is by allogeneic bone marrow transplantation. The highest rates of cure are achieved by transplantation during the chronic phase of the disorder, and are in the vicinity of 80%. They fall to 50–60% if transplantation is undertaken only after metamorphosis to acute leukemia. In the absence of a suitable donor for allogeneic transplantation this is one of the conditions where a single haplotype incompatible bone marrow donor transplant may be considered justifiable (Chapter 7).

DRUGS USED IN TREATMENT OF THE CHRONIC PHASE

The most commonly used agents are Hydroxyurea or Busulphan which is also called Myleran. Hydroxyurea is relatively non-toxic and is the agent of choice for initial therapy. Monitoring of blood counts at monthly intervals is desirable. Hydroxyurea cannot be used as the conditioning regimen for bone marrow transplantation. Recently a new biologic product known as alpha-interferon has also been shown to be useful in the treatment of the chronic phase. Busulphan in small daily doses is also relatively non-toxic, but more marrow suppressive than hydroxyurea. In very high doses Busulphan combined with cyclophosphamide is used as a conditioning regimen for bone marrow transplantation. Other conditioning regimens use total body irradiation in combination with cyclophosphamide and occasionally with additional Busulphan. In successfully treated patients the short and long term complications are those of the transplantation procedure (Chapter 7).

JUVENILE CHRONIC MYELOID LEUKEMIA AND MYELODYSPLASIA

These conditions most often present in early childhood or occasionally in teenage. Bruising and bleeding are prominent features as well as non-specific skin rashes. There is also often a tendency to infection. Almost always the spleen and liver are considerably enlarged. There may also be enlargement of lymph nodes. The blood count in juvenile chronic myeloid leukemia shows a relative increase of white cells but, in contrast to chronic myeloid leukemia, there is also often a low platelet count and anemia. In myelodysplasia all aspects of the blood count may be reduced. The bone marrow shows a reduction of platelet-producing cells. There is no Philadelphia chromosome but there may be other changes in the genetic material which confirm the diagnosis.

TREATMENT

These conditions can only be cured with bone marrow transplantation. When this is impossible then bleeding and infections are treated with platelet transfusion and antibiotics. Frequently the spleen grows to a very large size and surgical removal of the spleen may greatly improve the quality of the child's life. Death without therapeutic intervention is usually due to infection or hemorrhage. To ensure that death is as peaceful and painless as possible, it is best to treat hemorrhage with transfusion of platelets and infection with antibiotics. However, anemia is not treated with transfusions of red blood cells because death from anemia is more peaceful and dignified than that from hemorrhage or infection.

CHAPTER 13

Non-Hodgkin's Lymphoma (NHL)

These are malignancies of the cells of the immune system and are closely related to acute lymphocytic leukemia. The cells that are most frequently involved are the lymphocytes. Occasionally accessory cells of the immune system variously called histiocytes, macrophages or reticulum cells are also involved.

DIAGNOSIS

Unlike acute lymphocytic leukemia, the disease arises from the cells of the lymph nodes or the thymus. The thymus is an important immune regulating organ in front of the heart and is most active in childhood. As a result of the origin of this malignancy from the cells of the immune system, the presentation is usually with swelling of the lymph nodes. If there is appreciable swelling of the thymus then it can, by virtue of its size, compress certain structures in the chest particularly the windpipe (trachea) and the great veins returning blood from the upper part of the body. If this occurs, the patient will show swelling and redness of the face, and may be severely short of breath and have a dry cough. Occasionally these symptoms may be mistaken for asthma or croup.

Swelling of the lymph nodes of the abdomen may also present in deceptive ways. Sometimes the enlarged lymph nodes act as a focus for inversion of the inside of the bowel in a similar fashion to socks being inverted when folded. This is diagrammatically illustrated in Figure 15. The medical term for this is intussusception. At other times the enlarged glands may block

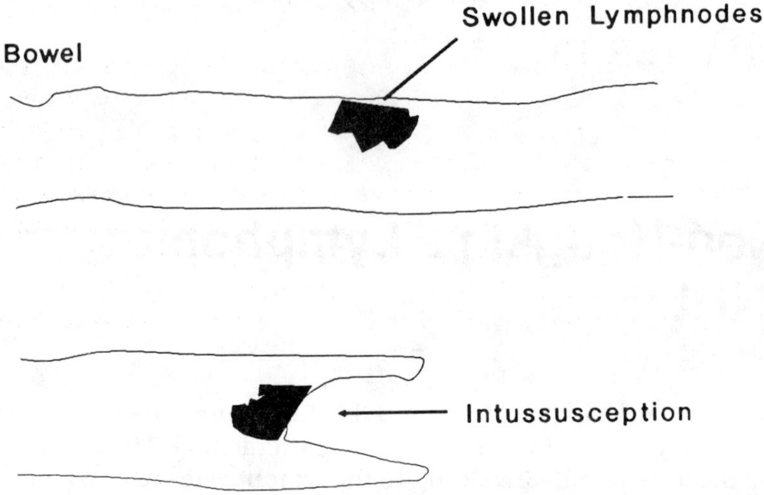

FIGURE 15 Intussusception. The swollen lymph nodes in the bowel wall act as the pivot for inversion of the bowel which is caused by the peristaltic movement of the bowel wall.

the bowel causing pain, vomiting and constipation. Occasionally enlargement of the glands results in production of excessive amounts of fluid in the abdominal cavity giving rise to a protuberant abdomen (ascites).

There are other rare modes of presentation but usually they are consequences of the effect of pressure on surrounding tissues.

STAGING

The diagnosis of non-Hodgkin's lymphoma is made by biopsy of the enlarged glands. At the same time, in most cases it is necessary to also perform a bone marrow aspirate and spinal tap. This is required because certain lymphomas also infiltrate the bone marrow and the central nervous systems. When this happens the condition is similar to ALL and is sometimes called the leukemia/lymphoma syndrome.

In addition to the above tests it will be necessary to assess the extent of other organ infiltration by x-ray, CT scan and ultrasound techniques. The liver, spleen, kidney, ovaries and testes are occasionally involved in this condition.

In planning treatment and considering the prognosis, it is very helpful to determine the type of cell that has been involved in the malignancy. This can be done by means of laboratory studies using highly specific (monoclonal) antibodies. As with the leukemias, there are certain chromosome abnormalities which are associated with various sub-types of non-Hodgkin's lymphoma. These can be identified by chromosome analysis.

A combination of clinical and laboratory staging is used to plan treatment, estimate the prognosis and classify these lymphomas.

CLASSIFICATION

There have been many, very complicated classifications of the lymphomas which suggests that none is entirely satisfactory. Certain useful generalizations can however help to understanding of these disorders.

1. In childhood all lymphomas are aggressive in their behavior and appearance under the microscope and are therefore classified as high grade.
2. Treatment of lymphomas which have characteristics of the "T" cells of the immune system is different to those which have "B" cell characteristics.
3. In general, "T" cell lymphomas present with primary disease above the diaphragm but very rarely with primary abdominal disease. "B" cell lymphomas most often present with primary abdominal disease, but may also present with enlarged lymph nodes above the diaphragm e.g. the neck or occasionally as primary disease in the brain.
4. All lymphomas involving enlargement of the thymus are of "T" cell origin and frequently involve the bone marrow and the central nervous system.

GENETIC CHANGES ASSOCIATED WITH NHL

The "B" cell lymphomas are associated with translocations of pieces of chromosome 8 to other chromosomes. The best documented are t8;14 t8;2 t8;22. At present there is no equivalent information for the "T" cell or histiocytic lymphomas.

PROGNOSTIC FACTORS

With vigorous and appropriate treatment, 70–90+% of children with lymphomas that have not involved the bone marrow or the central nervous system can be cured. In children with bone marrow infiltration some 50% can be cured, but in those with organ infiltration and central nervous system involvement the cure rate is far lower, being approximately 20%.

TREATMENT

Early Disease (Stage I or II)

This is usually defined as involvement of a single group of lymph nodes or the involvement of an organ with only its draining lymph nodes. It excludes involvement of the major lymph nodes in the chest and abdominal cavities. Stage I and II disease is curable with surgery and a short course of chemotherapy lasting some 6 months.

The chemotherapy consists of multiple drugs which are also used in the treatment of acute lymphocytic leukemia. They are usually given in higher doses than in leukemia. The two major regimens most often used are called by their acronyms of COMP (Cytoxan, Oncovin, Vincristine, Methotrexate, Prednisone) or CHOP (Cytoxan, hydroxydaunomycin, oncovin (vincristine), prednisone). In the case of non-abdominal primary tumors, it is also necessary to treat with a series of spinal taps using methotrexate to eliminate the possibility of infiltration of the central nervous system. In early stage abdominal lymphomas, infiltration of the central nervous system is so rare that a course of spinal taps is not required.

ADVANCED DISEASE

This is usually defined as any disease involving the thymus and the lymph nodes in the chest cavity; abdominal disease which is surgically not resectable; or abdominal disease which involves the liver and spleen in addition to the lymph nodes; or the presence of lymphoma above and below the diaphragm or in the bone marrow and central nervous system. It is usually graded as stage III or IV.

In most children at the time of presentation there is a large tumor cell mass. Immediate treatment with chemotherapy has a high chance of causing kidney damage by the breakdown product of the tumor cells. For this reason it is often wise to delay chemotherapy, meanwhile instituting treatment with intravenous fluids, and drugs which prevent blockage of the kidneys. In children with massive disease in the chest cavity there is the additional problem of obstruction of the windpipe (trachea) and the great vessels which return blood to the heart. It is often best to admit such children to an intensive care unit where respiratory support measures can be rapidly implemented in case of respiratory failure prior to tumor shrinkage by chemotherapy.

The major modality of treatment is high dose multi-agent chemotherapy given for 12 months. There is a variety of regimens which can be used, and each treatment center will follow its own well defined regimen.

In general the "T" cell lymphomas present with mass disease above the diaphragm and are treated with the same or similar chemotherapy as the most unfavorable acute lymphocytic leukemias. This includes spinal taps and irradiation of the brain. It has been conclusively shown that irradiation of the chest mass does not improve, and may even hinder, the chance of cure. In children with bone marrow involvement the treatment is continued for 2 years.

In children with "B" cell lymphoma who present with primary intra-abdominal disease, effective chemotherapy regimens use high doses of cytoxan, the anthracyclines, prednisone, vincristine, methotrexate and in some regimens additional agents such as the nitrosoureas and bleomycin. As with early stage disease these chemotherapy regimens are given various acronyms e.g. high dose CHOP, MACOP–B etc. In contrast with early stage intra-abdominal disease the advanced abdominal lymphomas have a significant incidence of central nervous system involvement and require a course of spinal taps, but not irradiation of the brain.

In children with the less common histologic subtypes of lymphomas, or in those with unusual presentations e.g. diffuse lymph node involvement and primary lymphoma of one organ only, the mainstay of treatment is one of the regimens used for the treatment of "B" cell disease. In the rare patient with primary disease of the central nervous system, spinal taps and irradiation of the brain and spinal cord are essential, as well as chemotherapy to prevent the spread of the lymphoma to organs outside the central nervous system. The chemotherapy in these patients is less intensive than in those with advanced lymphomas because spinal irradiation reduces tolerance to intensive chemotherapy. Sometimes in such situations, it may be better to delay irradiation of the brain and spinal cord for 6 months to allow administration of intensive chemotherapy.

TOXICITY OF CHEMOTHERAPY

There is no doubt that the intensity of the various chemotherapy regimens is such that there are many side effects. These are drug specific, general, and psychological.

Drug Specific

Most of the regimens use high or very high doses of drugs such as cytoxan, methotrexate or prednisone. In addition to suppression of marrow function, high dose cytoxan causes severe nausea and vomiting, and some form of anti vomiting treatment is essential to make the treatment tolerable. High dose cytoxan always causes early hair loss. A serious but preventable complication is inflammation of the bladder presenting as blood in the urine (hematuria). This can be prevented by intravenous fluids given before and after administration of cytoxan.

High dose methotrexate is potentially fatal unless there is adequate kidney and liver function, high urinary output is induced and its antidote, folinic acid, is administered according to set schedules. It can also cause numerous other side effects. These include nausea and vomiting; marked decrease in appetite; damage to the mucous membranes of the mouth and the gut; mouth ulcers; diarrhoea and marked weight loss; hepatitis causing jaundice; kidney damage; light sensitivity causing rashes or sunburn; and hair loss. Careful monitoring of methotrexate blood levels can prevent these side effects in the majority of patients.

High dose prednisone causes rapid weight gain mostly on the trunk and face. This may cause the appearance of striae (stretch marks) on the skin of the abdomen, buttocks and breasts. Occasionally there are other side effects such as transient diabetes and major mood changes leading to inappropriate behavior.

The side effects of vincristine and the anthracyclines have already been discussed in Chapter 10. Bleomycin, when used in high doses, can cause thickening of the interstitial tissues of the lung leading to shortness of breath. This side effect is only seen with high cumulative doses of bleomycin, and can be monitored by regular tests of respiratory function. Bleomycin at any dose can also cause pigmentation of the skin, particularly at sites of skin trauma such as scratch marks. This pigmentation is sometimes very similar in appearance to dirt marks on the skin, and attempts have been made to get rid of it by vigorous scrubbing. This, of course, irritates the skin further and increases the pigmentation.

General

There is an increased susceptibility to infections by a wide variety of organisms. It is therefore wise to take precautions against exposure to infections. These include:

1. avoidance of crowds,
2. checking that visitors to the home do not have obvious infections, or have been recently exposed to infections,
3. arranging with school authorities to contact the family if infectious diseases appear in the school,
4. seeking early medical attention for symptoms of an infection e.g. fever.

Psychological

The intensity of treatment in advanced disease, is such that it is often difficult for the child to return to a normal life during treatment. It is necessary to support the patient through this time by reminding them that the course of treatment is relatively short, and by arranging for breaks from the monotony of hospital life. In children who required a period of admission to an intensive care unit there may be more severe problems related to the fear of death, and resentment of the invasion of integrity of their body while desperately ill.

Such children need to express their fears and resentment and should be encouraged to do so by their parents and professional attendants. Sometimes psychiatric consultation is also required.

Hair loss lasts throughout the treatment course, and leads to changes in self image and esteem. Again it is necessary to stress the temporary nature of these changes and to support the child by averting situations in which they may be made to feel inferior in the company of their friends. Well-meaning invitations to teenage parties may prove disastrous if not sensitively handled. On the whole, children tend to prefer the company of others undergoing a similar form of treatment, and this should be encouraged as it is a very useful form of group therapy.

RELAPSE

This is always a very serious complication and the principles of treatment are very similar to those of ALL. In early stage disease, relapse is very rare and if it occurs, it usually manifests with features of advanced disease. In advanced disease, relapse usually shows up as a transformation to leukemia, or with an isolated relapse in the central nervous system or the testes.

In patients with early stage disease, change to one of the protocols used for treatment of advanced disease may prove curative. In those with advanced disease presenting as leukemia, allogeneic bone marrow transplantation offers the only chance of cure. With isolated relapses in patients who had bone marrow involvement at presentation but have no evidence of bone marrow involvement at relapse, irradiation and 12–24 months of different chemotherapy may prove effective. However, the relapse rate is so high that a preferable course of action is allogeneic transplantation. In the case of primary intra-abdominal disease of the "B" cell type without bone marrow involvement, autologous bone marrow transplantation is the preferred option. In patients with multiple relapses or a resistant central nervous system relapse, there is no chance of cure and, as with acute leukemia, treatment should be concerned with alleviating symptoms and concentrating attention on the quality of life.

CHAPTER 14

Hodgkin's Disease

This condition is a malignancy of the lymph nodes often associated with subtle abnormalities of the function of the immune system. It is eight times more common in boys. It differs from the non-Hodgkin's lymphomas in that, in Hodgkin's disease, the cell or cells of origin of the malignancy are as yet unknown and the rate of growth of the tumor is much slower.

DIAGNOSIS

The most common presentation is gradual enlargement of lymph nodes which eventually are noticed as a lump. Sometimes there is quite marked fluctuation in size of the lymph nodes. Usually, general health remains good but occasionally there is weight loss, night sweats and recurrent virus infections. The most frequent sites of involvement are the lymph nodes of the neck, but all other lymph node areas may also be involved. Of particular importance are the lymph nodes in the chest which can enlarge to the same extent as those with non-Hodgkin's lymphoma, with compression of the windpipe and the great vessels. There may also be involvement of certain organs of the body which are not considered to be part of the lymphatic system e.g. liver and lungs.

When there is a suspicion of Hodgkin's disease the diagnosis is established by a biopsy of the enlarged lymph nodes. This is a minor surgical procedure, and usually there is no need to excise all the involved glands.

STAGING

Frequently the extent of Hodgkin's disease is greater than is apparent by feeling for enlarged lymph nodes and organs of the body. The choice of the staging procedure is dependent on the treatment approach that will be used in the treatment center. In those treatment centers where radiation therapy is the main treatment modality, surgical staging will be required. This involves an exploration of the abdominal lymph nodes and removal of all or part of the spleen. This is called a staging laparotomy. There are major disadvantages to this type of staging because it involves a substantial surgical procedure, and removal of the spleen increases the risk of serious bacterial infections. In general there is a reluctance to use staging laparotomy in children.

In those centers that use chemotherapy as the mainstay of treatment, staging is undertaken by means of radiologic techniques and with nuclear isotopes, without recourse to surgery and in particular without splenectomy. This approach to staging of childhood Hodgkin's disease is gaining favor in the majority of childhood cancer treatment centers.

At the completion of staging procedures, it is possible to classify the disease according to the extent of tumor spread, the presence of symptoms of the disease and details of the microscopic appearance.

Stage I and II disease involves a single group of lymph nodes, or adjoining groups of nodes on the same side of the diaphragm and includes patients with involvement of the lymph nodes in the chest cavity. Stage III and IV disease involves lymph node groups on both sides of the diaphragm or involvement of nodes on the same side of the diaphragm and the liver. Disease involving lymph nodes on both sides of the diaphragm as well as liver and spleen is classified as stage IV, as is involvement of bone marrow and the lungs.

The severity of Hodgkin's disease is further classified according to whether there have been significant weight loss, night sweats and fever. If these symptoms are present the disease is called "B" type and if they are absent it is called "A" type.

The purpose of staging and the A and B classification is to help decide the intensity of treatment and the prognosis. The histological appearance of Hodgkin's disease is also a guide to prognosis. The best response to treatment occurs in patients with stage IA and IIA disease and the histological appearance of lymphocyte predominance or nodular sclerosis. Less favorable response to treatment occurs in patients with stage III and IV disease, B symptoms and the histological appearance of lymphocyte depletion or mixed cellularity.

Recently however, there has been such a marked improvement in the cure rate of Hodgkin's disease that staging and classification are of diminishing importance in assessing the chance of cure. Overall complete cure of Hodgkin's disease occurs in 80–90% of patients.

TREATMENT

The choice of the best treatment method is predominantly influenced by the undesirable long term side effects of treatment.

Irradiation

If this is used as the only treatment modality then there are 3 major consequences of that decision:

1. "Staging laparotomy" with some form of surgery on the spleen is mandatory.
2. The dose of irradiation will impair growth of the irradiated tissues. This leads to physical deformity. The younger the child the greater will be the extent of the deformity.
3. Depending on the dose of radiation the recurrence rate is 10–40%. In this case chemotherapy will be required for treatment and the patient will suffer the long term consequences of both treatment modalities.

Irradiation and Chemotherapy

If this treatment approach is used then:

1. Staging laparotomy is not required.
2. The dose and the field of irradiation can be reduced. This reduces but does not eliminate the long term consequences of physical deformity.

3. The recurrence rate is reduced to approximately 5–10% but the patient is exposed to the risks of the long term complications of both modalities of treatment. However, with reduced doses and fields of irradiation and shortened courses of chemotherapy, these risks are lower than when chemotherapy is used after irradiation had failed.

Chemotherapy

Chemotherapy has always been the treatment of choice of stage III and IV disease with cure rates of 60%. There have been studies from Uganda, the U.K. and Australia which have shown it to be even more effective in stage I and II disease. The major advantages are that a staging laparotomy is not required, and the patient is exposed to the side effects of only one treatment modality. The major side effects are those of the chemotherapeutic agents chosen for treatment. These are the probability of infertility in males and a small chance of acute myeloid leukemia.

CHEMOTHERAPY REGIMENS

There is a large variety of regimens in use but the best established ones are:

1. MOPP—Mustine (nitrogen mustard), oncovin (vincristine) Procarbazine, prednisone. One course consists of two injections of mustine and oncovin on days 1 and 8, and 14 days of procarbazine and prednisone taken by mouth.
2. ABVD—Adriamycin, bleomycin, vinblastine, DTIC. One course consists of 2 injections given on days 1 and 14.
3. ChlVPP—Chlorambucil, vinblastine, procarbazine and prednisone. One course consists of 14 days of chlorambucil, procarbazine and prednisone all given by mouth and 2 injections of vinblastine on days 1 and 8.

For early stage disease it is usual to use 3–4 courses, and for more advanced disease, 6 courses of chemotherapy.

New regimens which use agents with less potential for long term toxicity are currently under investigation.

IRRADIATION REGIMENS

These are mainly named in relation to the extent of irradiation. Those with the smallest field of irradiation are called *involved field*. Those which encompass adjoining groups of lymph nodes are called *extended field*. Those which irradiate all lymph nodes areas above the diaphragm are called *mantle*, while those below the diaphragm are called *inverted Y*.

RELAPSE

The most resistant types of disease are those with lung involvement and marked enlargement of the lymph nodes in the chest cavity. In such patients there may be only partial response at the completion of therapy using either chemotherapy or irradiation. It is sometimes necessary to wait for some time to see whether this partial response represents slow resolution of scar tissue which is a feature of certain types of Hodgkin's disease, or whether there is persistence of active Hodgkin's disease. If active Hodgkin's disease remains it will progress.

In the presence of active disease, treatment is changed to another modality e.g. from chemotherapy to irradiation. Unfortunately response is usually poor, with progression of the disease. There is a variety of experimental chemotherapy regimens which can be used under these circumstances, and in some instances autologous marrow rescue with massive doses of chemotherapy has been attempted. Overall the results have been disappointing.

COMPLICATIONS OF TREATMENT

These are best considered according to modality of treatment and classified according to whether they occur in the first 6–12 months (early) or between 10–20 years (late).

Chemotherapy

Early complications include nausea and vomiting, discomfort with injections, effects on the blood count which may require postponement of treatment and transfusions. If transfusions are required, the blood products should be first irradiated to prevent the uncommon but very real possibility of graft versus host disease. Infections, particularly shingles (Herpes Zoster) may occur after treatment has ceased.

Late complications—In boys who have reached puberty and received 6 courses of MOPP, there is a high probability of infertility. It is not known whether the infertility is permanent or temporary. Infertility does not occur in girls because their ova are already formed at birth. It is claimed that infertility is less common with ABVD, but the statistics are less complete than those for MOPP.

In boys who have not commenced puberty or have only just entered puberty, and in all those boys who have received only 3–4 courses of MOPP, there is a lower chance of infertility but its precise incidence is unknown.

In all chemotherapy treated patients, there is a small risk of developing leukemia. In those treated with at least 6 courses of MOPP the incidence is approximately 4%. In those treated with 3–4 courses of MOPP or other chemotherapy regimens the incidence is unknown but is likely to be less than 4%.

Irradiation

Early complications—Irradiation is usually well tolerated apart from a propensity to infection, including shingles. In cases where irradiation and chemotherapy are combined there may be more side effects from irradiation because the chemotherapy compounds the cell damage caused by irradiation. In such cases there may be inflammation of skin and mucous membranes such as those of the esophagus giving rise to difficulty in swallowing.

Late complications—There is arrest of growth of the irradiated tissues which results in uneven growth. If the irradiation was given as a mantle in children who have not finished growing, then typically there is a thin neck and underdevelopment of the lower jaw, hollow appearance of the upper part of the shoulders and a small chest. If the irradiation was given as an inverted Y then the abdominal cavity is similarly affected, resulting in a small and narrow pelvis and often unstable hips. These body deformities may result in difficulty in forming relationships with the opposite sex.

There are also more specific complications which are related to long-term effects of irradiation on certain body organs. In the neck there may be impairment of thyroid function. In the chest there may be thickening of the lungs or the membranes around the heart. Occasionally the blood vessels supplying the heart are thickened resulting in early onset of coronary heart disease. In the abdomen there may be inflammation and polyps of the bladder and damage to the hip bones.

There is an increased risk of late cancers both of the benign and malignant types. These involve the thyroid gland, muscles and soft tissues, bone and, in females, breast. Leukemia is a rare complication of irradiation alone but when irradiation and chemotherapy are combined, it may occur in as many as 14% of patients.

Infertility is not a complication of irradiation unless it is necessary to directly irradiate the testes or the ovaries.

CONCLUSION

Despite the depressingly long list of possible complications, they are all rare, and the child with Hodgkin's disease has an excellent chance of being completely cured. Chemothcrapy avoids the profound possible effects on physical appearance, and therefore provides the least undesirable long term side effects.

CHAPTER 15

Wilms' Tumor (Nephroblastoma)

This is a malignancy of primitive embryonal cells which normally form the kidneys. Rarely, the tumor is associated with other congenital malformations such as marked asymmetry of one side of the body with or without abnormalities of the eye. In these instances there is loss of genetic material on the short arm of chromosome 11. In the much more common tumors without other associated abnormalities, there are also fine structural changes in a similar region of chromosome 11. The significance of these findings is its demonstration of the close link between tumor formation and certain errors in cell proliferation during development of the embryo.

DIAGNOSIS

The most common mode of presentation is with a prominent lump in the child's abdomen. This is usually first noticed by a parent and confirmed by a medical examination.

Less common presentations are painless passing of blood in the urine, the presence of very high blood pressure or sudden severe abdominal pain with shock due to the rupture of a very large tumor.

There is often difficulty in distinguishing between Wilms' tumor and a more malignant tumor of the adrenal gland which is situated just above the kidney, and is known as neuroblastoma. In most instances this difficulty is resolved by the use of ultrasound or CAT scans which shows the site of origin of the tumor.

STAGING

Some of the staging is undertaken prior to surgery but most occurs during surgery. Wilms' tumor most often spreads to the lungs, and a chest x-ray prior to surgery will reveal any metastases. If there is suspicion of their presence, or if the chest x-ray shows one or more metastases, a CAT scan of the lungs is required to more accurately determine their number and distribution. In most patients the tumor is deemed resectable, and further staging is undertaken during surgery and by the pathologist when examining the tumor under the microscope.

Stage I and II: These are tumors within the confines of the kidney capsule; have not infiltrated into surrounding tissues such as liver or the diaphragm; have not involved the regional lymph nodes; and have not ruptured before or during surgery.

Stage III, IV and V: Those with local extension or rupture are stage III while those with distant spread are stage IV. When both kidneys are involved the tumor is stage V.

In a small number of patients the tumor is deemed inoperable, usually because of its massive size with or without infiltration of neighboring organs, or because both kidneys are involved. Such tumors are always stage III, IV or V. It is usually wise to obtain a biopsy of the tumor prior to proceeding with treatment. The biopsy confirms the diagnosis and allows pathological staging.

PATHOLOGY CLASSIFICATION

Wilms' tumor is one of the few solid tumors of childhood where the microscopic features are strongly associated with response to treatment. These are classified into favorable and unfavorable histology. Approximately 90% of Wilms' tumors have the favorable histology with predominance of primitive cells which normally give rise to mature kidney tissue. In 10% the predominant cells have features of other cells, such as primitive muscle cells, or supporting tissue and these are called unfavorable histology Wilms' tumors.

TREATMENT

The major modalities are surgery, chemotherapy and in a small number of complicated cases, irradiation. The treatment of the tumor has been well defined by successive and well-planned National Wilms' tumor studies in the USA as well as by European multinational studies.

For stage I and II tumors with favorable histology, cure rates close to 100% are achieved with surgical excision of the tumor followed by a short course of chemotherapy using vincristine and actinomycin–D. No irradiation is required.

For stage III tumors the strategy of treatment depends on whether the tumor is initially thought to be operable. Operable tumors are treated with irradiation to the tumor bed and chemotherapy with vincristine and actinomycin–D for 12–15 months.

One of the major problems with stage III tumors however, is tumor rupture before surgery or spill of tumor during surgery due to its size and the extent of infiltration. In such instances it will be necessary to irradiate the whole abdominal cavity. This is far more toxic than tumor bed irradiation because of the need to irradiate most of the bowel. This causes poor appetite and reduced absorption of food. A period of intravenous feeding may be required to overcome this toxicity. Late complications include increased susceptibility to formation of scar tissue between loops of bowel which may cause bowel obstruction, and a theoretical risk of later second cancers of organs of the abdominal cavity.

In patients considered inoperable and increasingly more often in those whose clinical findings and investigations show a stage III tumor, chemotherapy is used as initial treatment. It is often so effective in shrinking the tumor that it becomes removable without the risk of tumor spill. Sometimes the chemotherapy is so effective that at surgery the stage III situation has changed to stage I or II, and there may even be debate on whether tumor bed irradiation is necessary. In most cases without preoperative tumor rupture, preoperative chemotherapy will prevent the need for total abdominal irradiation and restrict it to the tumor bed only.

In patients with stage IV tumors, chemotherapy usually consists of vincristine, actinomycin–D and adriamycin. There is often complete disappearance of lung lesions with this chemotherapy and at the completion of treatment the CT scan is normal. In those patients in whom there are residual lesions after adequate chemotherapy, surgical excision will achieve a cure. Irradiation of the lungs should be avoided and used only in those rare instances where chemotherapy and adequate surgery have failed to eradicate the tumor in the lungs, or where new tumors have appeared despite chemotherapy. With this approach to treatment the cure rate in favorable histology stage IV Wilms' tumor is approximately 80%.

In patients with bilateral tumors (Stage V) the major challenge is to preserve sufficient normal kidney tissue to allow survival with normal kidney function. In recent years it has become apparent that this aim can be achieved by using preoperative chemotherapy as described above, and by carefully planned surgical approach aiming to excise only those parts of the kidneys which still appear abnormal. There is nothing to be gained from the old approach of excising the most involved kidney and part of the least involved kidney as the first step in treatment, because this approach fails to preserve as much normal kidney tissue as possible.

UNFAVORABLE HISTOLOGY

The 10% of patients with this type of tumor have the worst outlook and most deaths from Wilms' tumor occur among them. They often have unusual presentations and are almost always stage III or IV. The metastases may be more widespread and involve the bones as well as lungs. The mainstay of treatment is intensive chemotherapy with regimens which use drugs such as cis-platinum, the epipodophyllotoxin (VP–16) and an analog of cytoxan such as ifosfamide. There is still insufficient experience with this type of approach to determine whether it will improve the very poor outlook for this uncommon form of Wilms' tumor.

COMPLICATIONS OF TREATMENT

These are mainly the side effects of chemotherapy such as nausea and vomiting, depression of bone marrow and immune function, and hair loss. Usually they are mild. Actinomycin–D may cause a skin rash which can be severe and may preclude its further use. It also accentuates the effect of irradiation, and the timing of actinomycin D in relation to irradiation particularly in the region of the liver must be carefully planned. It is unwise to use actinomycin–D within 6 weeks of irradiation.

Adriamycin can also accentuate the effects of irradiation but its major toxicity is to heart muscle when a cumulative dose of 400mg/m2 has been exceeded. Where irradiation of the lungs is required, the dose of adriamycin should not exceed 300mg/m2.

Tumor bed irradiation is usually well tolerated, and apart from retardation of growth of tissues in the irradiation bed it has few complications.

CONCLUSION

Wilms' tumor of favorable histology is eminently curable even when the tumor is disseminated or involves both kidneys. The approach to treatment is directed at achieving a cure with the least possible long term complications. However, the outlook for unfavorable histology Wilms' tumor remains poor.

CHAPTER 16

Neuroblastoma

The nervous system may be subdivided in two major components—somatic and autonomic. The somatic system regulates and controls most of the voluntary motor functions e.g. walking and writing. The autonomic system regulates involuntary functions such as control of blood pressure, heart rate, bowel and bladder tone. The sympathetic autonomic nervous system has nerve cells which are situated outside the spinal cord and extend from the neck to the pelvis. In the abdomen these nerve cells are situated in nerve cell centers close to the major blood vessels and in glands known as the adrenal glands which are situated just above the kidneys. The distribution of the nerve cells of the sympathetic autonomic nervous system is shown in Figure 16.

Neuroblastoma is a malignancy of the primitive cells that normally differentiate to form cells of the sympathetic autonomic nervous system. The malignancy may arise from any of the cells that extend from the neck to the pelvis including those of the adrenal glands. The neuroblastoma cells have often matured to some extent, and they produce chemicals which are part of the metabolic pathways of adrenaline production. These chemicals are excreted in the urine and can be accurately measured.

The behavior of these malignant cells appears to be strongly influenced by the age of the child and by the site of origin of the tumor. In general the best outlook for cure is in the youngest children and in tumors arising outside the abdominal cavity.

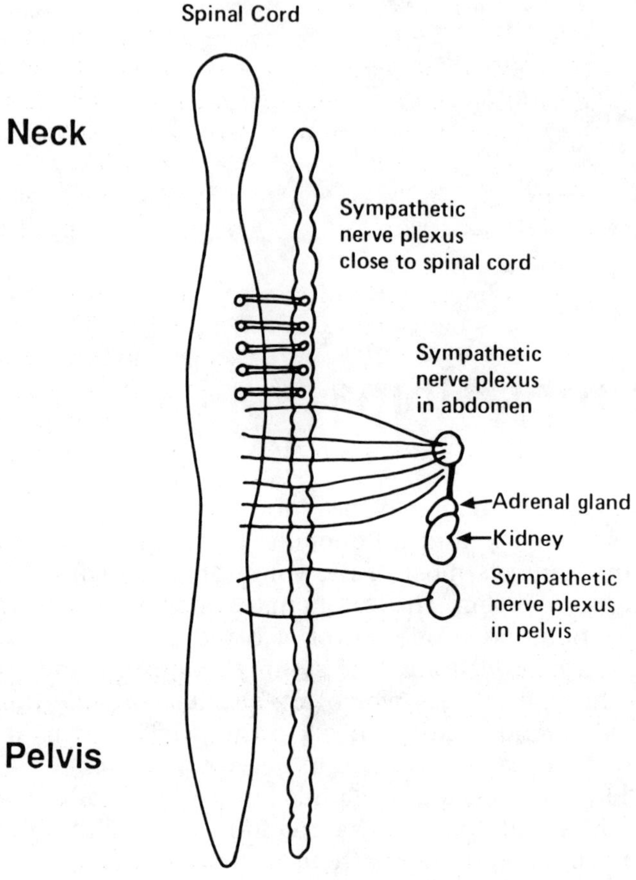

FIGURE 16 The sympathetic autonomic nervous system.

DIAGNOSIS

Neuroblastoma can mimic many diseases and it is therefore difficult to diagnose it early in the course of the illness. The nerve cells from which the tumor arises are situated at sites which cannot be readily felt and therefore the tumor can grow to a very large size before it becomes clinically obvious. In addition neuroblastoma cells have an innate tendency to migrate from their site of origin to other parts of the body, particularly the bone marrow, the bones, lymph nodes and tissue at the back the eyes. The growth of neuroblastoma at these sites may be the first manifestation of the tumor. Growth of neuroblastoma in bone marrow and bones mimics leukemia. Enlargement of lymph nodes may mimic lymphomas or infection, while growth in the tissues behind the eyes may cause them to become prominent and this may be mistaken as a manifestation of thyroid disease.

The most common mode of presentation is with abdominal pain, distension, poor appetite and weight loss. There is often a lump on the skull, enlarged lymph nodes, pallor and protrusion of one or both eyes. Medical examination reveals a large craggy abdominal lump. Special investigations are then undertaken usually consisting of abdominal CAT scans, bone scans, bone marrow tests and collection of urine to measure the products of adrenaline metabolism. Some of the ones most commonly measured are called methylhydroxy mandelic acid (MHMA), Homovanilic acid (HVA), dopamine, adrenaline and nor-adrenaline. The urine test is very helpful in monitoring response to treatment.

The above presentation is typical of advanced tumors particularly those arising from the abdomen and accounts for at least 80% of all patients with neuroblastoma. Tumors arising from sites other than the abdomen have a better outlook and often present with distinct features. Those arising in the neck may present with asymmetric size of pupils and a lump in the upper portion of the neck. Those arising in the chest are often accidentally noticed on a routine chest x-ray. Those arising in the pelvis may press on the bladder and rectum causing retention of urine and constipation. Sometimes these relatively benign tumors may be complicated by growth of the tumor into the spinal canal. When this happens there may be spinal cord compression leading to paraplegia. This type of complication is more common with pelvic than thoracic or neck tumors. It constitutes an emergency situation requiring prompt surgery on the spinal canal to relieve pressure on the spinal cord.

In children under the age of 1 year and often in infants under the age of 6 months there is another characteristic presentation which, while it appears alarming, is in fact associated with a good outcome. This is called the stage IVS presentation. Attention is drawn to the infant by the appearance of multiple lumps under the skin which have a blue tinge. Often these infants also have abdominal distention.

The diagnosis of neuroblastoma is established when the condition has been thought of and its presence confirmed by special investigations. If there is infiltration of the bone marrow then a marrow aspirate together with the measurement of adrenaline products excreted in the urine will establish the diagnosis. If marrow infiltration is not present then in the majority of centers a biopsy of the tumor is undertaken. In some centers however, the presence of a tumor lump and raised levels of adrenaline products are considered sufficient for diagnosis.

STAGING

Initial investigations are directed at diagnosis and staging.

Stage I – These are tumors which can be totally excised.

Stage II – Those which after excision leave a residue of tumor in their vicinity.

Stage III – Those which cannot be excised because of their size or anatomical location such as proximity to major blood vessels or because of regional lymph node involvement.

Stage IV – Those which have spread to distant parts of the body.

Stage IVS – These are tumors in infants where there is a small adrenal primary and wide spread metastases including the skin and liver but no involvement of bone.

Recently convincing evidence has been accumulated to show that a high content and expression of an oncogene known as N–myc is associated with advanced disease.

PROGNOSTIC FACTORS

The most important indicators of a favorable outcome of the illness are the age and the stage of the disease.

Age

The most favorable outcome is seen in children less than one year of age while that in children between the ages of 1–2 years is intermediate. Children over the age of 10 years also have a moderately better outlook but this is mainly for prolonged survival rather than cure.

Stage

Early stages (stage I and II) of the disease have an 80–90% chance of cure in all age groups. Unfortunately these stages are only common in very young children. Stage IVS which virtually always occurs in children under the age of 1 year, has an 80% chance of spontaneous cure. Virtually the only mortality in infants with stage IVS disease occurs in those with massive liver infiltration which prevents movement of the diaphragm and thus interferes with breathing. Stage III disease is far less favorable and occurs more often in children older than one year. The chance of cure is almost entirely dependent on the ability to shrink the tumor with treatment so that it becomes operable. Cures in stage III disease occur in approximately 40%. Stage IV disease is unfortunately the most common form of presentation and has a very grave prognosis, with cures in less than 5% of children. The content and expression of the oncogene N–myc is strongly related to disease outcome. Increased levels of N–myc indicate a poor chance of cure.

TREATMENT

Nature has set a model for the best treatment of this malignancy, namely the spontaneous resolution of stage IVS neuroblastoma. Infants with this condition may be riddled with metastases, yet over a period of months these disappear spontaneously. Their disappearance is associated with microscopic features of maturation of the malignant cells to normal nerve cells. It is as if there occurred a belated "switch on" of genetic information which stopped the cells from aberrant behavior and "tuned" them into normal autonomic nerve cell behavior and habitat. Researchers are investigating the mechanisms of this series of events. Hope for cure lies in research on these mechanisms.

Meanwhile the only truly curative approach to neuroblastoma is surgical excision. This is possible in stage I and II disease and is the only form of treatment required. In some centers surgical excision of the adrenal primary site in stage IVS neuroblastoma is also recommended because occasionally these primary sites may revert to malignant behavior.

In patients with stage III disease it is normal to use some form of chemotherapy to attempt to shrink the tumor. The drugs which are mainly used are the anthracyclines, the alkylating agents and cis-platinum. It is rational in these patients to consider the use of very high dose chemotherapy and autologous bone marrow transplantation to reduce the tumor to an operable size. In some centers, particularly in France chemotherapy is supplemented with irradiation, but this approach makes subsequent surgery more difficult.

There is a great variety of chemotherapy regimens to the treatment of stage IV disease. Their very number attests to their lack of effectiveness. In general they use the same drugs as outlined for stage III disease and are effective in alleviating pain and reducing the size of tumor, but not in curing the child. Many centers attempt to consolidate on the gains of standard dose chemotherapy by using very high doses of chemotherapy with autologous and, less often, allogeneic bone marrow transplantation. Autologous transplantation is relatively harmless and may prolong life without excessive suffering. Allogeneic transplantation with conditioning treatment consisting of multiple chemotherapeutic agents and total body irradiation is extremely hazardous and associated with severe and prolonged sickness. It is therefore difficult to justify except in the most unusual circumstances e.g. complete and stable disappearance of all signs of stage IV disease and the availability of a well-matched sibling donor.

ADVICE ON ATTITUDES TO TREATMENT

There is no doubt that treatment of stage I, II and III neuroblastoma is essential to achieve a cure and is effective in virtually all patients with stage I and II disease and many stage III patients. Stage IVS disease should not be overtreated with chemotherapy or irradiation because of the high probability of spontaneous resolution.

The main problem arises in stage IV disease where treatment does not offer cure. The family must balance the advantages and disadvantages of treatment bearing in mind the low chance of cure. Treatment that is effective in alleviating the symptoms of the tumor and in prolonging life is clearly desirable, but frequently there is pressure to go beyond this. The decision is always difficult because of the natural tendency of many parents to accept even the most slender chance of cure as better than none at all. The decision to undertake experimental treatment may severely impair the quality of the child's remaining life because of the nature of side effects of therapy and prolonged hospitalization. In making the decision it is essential to consider the proposed treatment method entirely from the point of view of the patient i.e. the child. Experience in treating adults with advanced cancer suggests that the majority prefer death at home and with dignity rather than in hospital following intensive treatment.

LONG TERM COMPLICATIONS

These are uncommon. The one of major significance is curvature of the spine in those children who required spinal canal surgery to relieve pressure of the tumor on the spinal cord. Removal of one adrenal gland has no long term consequences and replacement treatment with hormones is not required.

NON-MEDICAL APPROACHES TO TREATMENT

In patients with stage IV disease who are incurable there is a tendency to seek cures outside the realm of scientific medicine. In the experience of the author and his colleagues there has not been a cure from non-medical approaches in true stage IV neuroblastoma. As with medical treatment, the deterioration of the quality of life imposed on the child by non-medical methods of treatment will in all probability markedly diminish enjoyment of life, if only because it constantly reminds the child that they are sick and therefore different to other children. In youth it is possible to temporarily forget even the most unpleasant facts and so, in the face of a terminal illness, to still snatch moments of pleasure. This should not be denied to a child with incurable neuroblastoma, in exchange for a non-existent chance of a "miracle" cure.

CHAPTER 17

Bone Tumors

There are two main types of malignant tumors that have their origin from the cells that give rise to bone and its external lining, the periosteum. These tumors are called osteosarcoma and Ewing's tumor. Osteosarcomas are distinguished from Ewing's tumor by the greater maturity of osteosarcoma cells which deposit bone tissue (osteoid) in their immediate environment. In some instances, there are additional microscopic features which lead to a different label for some of these tumors which are named after prominent microscopic features e.g. fibrohistiocytoma, osteoblastic, chondroblastic or telangiectatic osteosarcomas. Despite these different names they are all malignant tumors of the osteosarcoma type.

It has been known for a long time that a small proportion of osteosarcomas are caused by irradiation of bone, and that there is a far higher incidence of osteosarcoma in patients with an eye tumor known as retinoblastoma, than in the population in general. Recently it has been shown that subtle changes on chromosome 13 are associated with retinoblastoma and osteosarcoma. It is considered likely that in the future, an osteosarcoma gene site will be found on chromosome 13 and its characterization will considerably enhance our understanding of this tumor.

There have been studies to investigate the possibility that trauma to bone may initiate osteosarcoma, but none has shown any relationship between injury and tumor development.

In contrast to osteosarcoma, the malignant cells of Ewing's tumor show no differentiation and their environment has few distinguishing characteristics. There is no evidence that Ewing's tumor can be induced by radiation, or that it is associated with any other childhood tumor. There is also no evidence that it is induced by trauma.

Recently a chromosome translocation between chromosome 11 and 22 has been associated with Ewing's sarcoma. This is a very useful aid to confirmation of diagnosis of the tumor. The mechanism whereby this translocation confers malignant behavior on the cells is not yet known.

DIAGNOSIS AND STAGING

The most common presentation is lump and limp. The lump represents the tumor of the bone and it is often painful and hence the limp. In general, in osteosarcoma there is less pain than in Ewing's sarcoma. Osteosarcoma mostly involves the long bones of the lower limbs and the upper part of the upper arm, and occasionally the pelvis. Ewing's sarcoma may involve the same sites but may also involve the bones of the spinal column, ribs, shoulder girdle and skull. Osteosarcoma usually occurs in teenage and adolescence and is rare in young children. Ewing's sarcoma occurs in young as well as older children.

It is common to find that at the first presentation for medical attention the lump and limp are considered to be due to trauma, but eventually an x-ray of the painful site is ordered and it shows that the swelling is due to a tumor. The x-ray findings may suggest the possible nature of the tumor, but do not establish the diagnosis with certainty. In some patients with Ewing's sarcoma, the x-ray findings may be very similar to those of the bone infection known as osteomyelitis.

When there is a suspicion that a bone tumor is present it is wise to undertake staging before biopsy. Accurate staging requires radiographs and CAT scans of the limbs and the lungs, and an isotope bone scan to determine whether the tumor is confined to one area of the bone, or whether it has "skipped" along the bone, or involved multiple bones. Tumors can thus be staged as confined to their bone of origin or disseminated with metastases to other bones and/or lungs.

The precise nature of the tumor is determined by a biopsy. It is unwise to undertake both a biopsy and surgical excision of the tumor at the same time. The surgeon undertaking the biopsy has to plan and perform it in such a way that the chance of breaking the bone (fracture) is minimized. Despite careful precautions to avoid a fracture it may sometimes happen spontaneously, or with biopsy. The occurrence of such a fracture makes management of the tumor more difficult, but does not prejudice the chances of cure.

PROGNOSIS

There is a variety of factors which influence prognosis. The most important is vigorous treatment and this will be discussed later. Provided that the best treatment methods are available, there is a far better outlook in tumors confined to the bone of origin than in those which have spread to other organs. Spread to other bones has a worse prognosis than spread to the lungs. Tumors of the pelvis have the worst outlook despite very vigorous treatment. The treatment regimens most often used are designed to test the sensitivity of the tumor cells to chemotherapy. Sensitive tumors have clearly a better outlook than resistant ones. In osteosarcoma of the long bones which is sensitive to chemotherapy, a cure rate of 80–90% can be expected. In nonsensitive tumors the cure rate is in the vicinity of 30–50%. In pelvic osteosarcoma the cure rate is much lower at about 10–20%. In disseminated osteosarcoma involving other bones, cures are rare, but if only lungs are involved there is a 30% chance of cure.

In Ewing's sarcoma confined to one bone and sensitive to chemotherapy, a cure rate of 70–80% can be expected. In nonsensitive tumors the cure rate is approximately 40%. In pelvic Ewing's sarcoma cures are rare, and they are also rare in tumors that have disseminated to other bones. Tumors arising from the ribs, spinal column and skull have a 60–80% chance of cure.

In both tumors, relapse during treatment carries a poor prognosis except in the occasional cases when the only site of relapse is the lung. Relapse after treatment has ceased also has a poor prognosis, but again, if the relapse is confined to the lungs, there is a 20–30% chance of cure.

TREATMENT STRATEGIES

Planning a strategy of treatment which involves surgery, chemotherapy and irradiation is critical for successful treatment of these tumors.

In both tumors, chemotherapy given before surgery, or in some forms of Ewing's sarcoma before irradiation to the primary site, is the major form of treatment, and has dramatically increased the chances of cure. In the case of osteosarcoma there was some doubt expressed about the value of chemotherapy from one prominent treatment center (Mayo Clinic). This resulted in a clinical trial, in which, those patients who agreed to participate were randomly allocated to receive or not receive chemotherapy. The results in the chemotherapy treated group were clearly superior. Similarly, historical comparisons showed much better results since the introduction of chemotherapy in the treatment of osteosarcoma. On these grounds there can now be no rational argument against the use of chemotherapy in this tumor.

The approach to treatment also involves close cooperation and planning with a team of orthopedic surgeons (bone surgeons). It is the orthopedic surgeon who makes the decisions on the treatment of the tumor in the bone. The aim of surgery should be to remove the tumor with the involved segment of bone and a small surrounding margin of normal tissues without amputating the limb. This is called limb preservation. In experienced surgical hands this is often possible, but for the procedure to be technically feasible, without having to operate through cancer tissues, shrinkage of the tumor with chemotherapy is essential. It is necessary for the patient and the family to understand the importance of this type of approach to treatment in order for them to cope with the heavy stresses of pre-operative chemotherapy and the waiting period for major surgery.

In some patients with Ewing's sarcoma involving bones of the spinal column and skull, surgery is not possible. Even in these circumstances chemotherapy before irradiation is the correct strategy of treatment because irradiation is most effective when the tumor mass has been thus reduced to its minimum size.

In Ewing's tumor there is still some dispute about the value of surgery as compared to irradiation. The incontrovertible facts are that with irradiation there is: approximately a 30% chance of local tumor recurrence; complete arrest of growth of the irradiated bone; a small but definite risk of fracture of the bone; and a small but definite chance of inducing a second cancer such as osteosarcoma. Where it is possible to use surgery to preserve the limb, these risks are eliminated and surgery is therefore the better option. In some instances surgery is possible, but complete excision of tumor cannot be achieved because the tumor has infiltrated widely outside the confines of the bone and the periosteum. In such instances irradiation is given to the tumor site after surgery. Because most of the tumor has been surgically removed, the dose of irradiation is relatively small and this reduces its long term consequences. If surgery is entirely impossible (e.g. spinal column and skull) then irradiation is the only option.

The difficult choice is one between irradiation and amputation. Fortunately with modern surgical techniques this is becoming an increasingly uncommon event. Faced with such a choice it is important to remember that with irradiation these will be arrest of growth and weakness of the bone and limb. Sometimes an amputation with a good prosthesis is a better option than a poorly functioning limb which could be a site of Ewing's recurrence or the development of an osteosarcoma in 10–20 years time.

Pelvic tumors whether osteosarcoma or Ewing's present a particularly difficult problem. In these tumors there is usually substantial extension of the tumor outside the bone into the muscle lining the inside of the pelvic bones, and sometimes even into pelvic structures such as the bladder. Chemotherapy will usually shrink the tumor outside the bone but will not kill the tumor cells inside the bone. Irradiation has proven to be ineffective in controlling such bone tumors. The only chance for cure is surgery which entails complete excision of the tumor bearing bone. This type of surgery can be mutilating and may require the removal of the whole limb and half of the pelvis. There is a very natural tendency to recoil from such massive and deforming surgery and to prefer less drastic measures such as partial excision and irradiation at a lower dose. Unfortunately, in the case of pelvic tumors such an approach is very seldom successful in curing the patient. It may, under such circumstances be necessary to make the very hard decision to undertake massive surgery and accept the disabilities that result from it. It is sometimes helpful to compare this situation to a motor car accident with life threatening crush injuries to the limb and pelvis where there would be little hesitation to amputate in order to save life.

CHEMOTHERAPY

For both tumors it is usual to use multiple agents as intensively as possible.

Osteosarcoma

In this tumor a widely used regimen is known as high dose methotrexate (HDMTX) with folinic acid rescue. In this regimen, lethal doses of methotrexate are given and the normal cells are rescued with folinic acid. There are complicated biochemical reasons why folinic acid rescues normal cells more efficiently than tumor cells. There is a fine balance between the blood level of methotrexate and the time that the cells are exposed to these blood levels, and the ability to rescue with folinic acid. Factors affecting this balance have been accurately defined and specialized oncology centers employ one or another of these treatment protocols. It is essential to observe, with meticulous care, all details of such protocols because errors or omissions may have fatal consequences. These protocols require administration of set amounts and types of intravenous fluids, and measurements of kidney and liver function at set intervals, as well as blood levels of methotrexate. The response of the patient may vary from one treatment course to the next and regular monitoring is essential to forestall unexpected toxicity, and to take appropriate measures to deal with it.

Other drugs which have been shown to have a beneficial effect in osteosarcoma are adriamycin, cis-platinum, actinomycin–D, bleomycin and cytoxan.

In general, protocols for osteosarcoma utilize the most active agents for the particular patient. Some are designed to test tumor sensitivity to HDMTX prior to definitive surgery and, if the tumor is sensitive, continue the use of HDMTX. If the tumor is insensitive to HDMTX, chemotherapy is changed to predominant use of adriamycin and cis-platinum. Other protocols use adriamycin and cis-platinum from the beginning and continue these agents with or without HDMTX after definitive surgery.

The use of cis-platinum requires the same attention to details of administration as HDMTX. Cis-platinum can be toxic to kidneys, can impair hearing, and reduces the body levels of magnesium. Regular monitoring of its effects is essential for its safe use, and replacement of magnesium by taking oral preparations between courses is required. The combined use HDMTX and cis-platinum is particularly hazardous because both agents can cause serious kidney damage.

Rejection of Chemotherapy

Because of the unpleasant side effects of these chemotherapeutic agents and the frequent occurrence of osteosarcoma in teenagers and adolescents, tolerance to treatment is often poor. It is quite common for the patient to develop such dread of chemotherapy that they work out elaborate subterfuges to avoid or to postpone it. In some instances there is flat refusal to proceed with treatment. These crises are best handled by patient and sympathetic listening to the patient's complaints and rectification of minor details which often cause disproportionate annoyance. The patients' peers, and health staff not directly connected with chemotherapy are asked to help by listening to complaints, and by sympathetic encouragement. Pressure must be brought to bear to continue with treatment, and in the majority such an approach is successful and chemotherapy can proceed.

Chemotherapy of Ewing's Sarcoma

The chemotherapy of Ewing's sarcoma is also based on the use of multiple agents, but HDMTX and cis-platinum are not of particular value in this tumor. While most protocols employ a variety of agents always including cytoxan and adriamycin, there is growing evidence that a new drug, known as ifosfamide is of particular value. Another agent which is also active against this tumor is VP–16. The use of combinations of ifosfamide and VP–16 in Ewing's sarcoma may prove to be of substantial benefit.

SURGERY

In both tumors there is evidence that chemotherapy alone cannot eliminate all tumor cells from bone. When chemotherapy has reduced the tumor size, surgery is undertaken on the involved bone. The orthopedic surgeons in the majority of pediatric cancer centers are well aware of the new methods which allow excision of bone without amputation, and can choose the appropriate procedure by using either metal and ceramic inserts or, preferably bone transfer from one site to another.

While these procedures are amazingly successful in preserving limbs, they also involve a prolonged and often difficult period of rehabilitation during which the patient may need to be attached to external splints, or encased in heavy plaster casts. Intensive physiotherapy and great care with the use of the limb are always required. During this period of rehabilitation, chemotherapy is given at regular intervals. It is not easy to cope with all the events of this postoperative phase, and to do so, it is necessary to mobilize all sources of assistance that are available to the family.

Introduction of foreign materials to replace bone has with it the risk of infection. This is markedly aggravated by chemotherapy. Even trivial infections of the skin may result in severe infections at the site of the foreign material. Early antibiotic treatment, often intravenous, may be required for apparently trivial infections.

In addition to limb surgery, operation on the lungs may be vital for the treatment of osteosarcoma that has spread to the lungs. Surgery on the lungs is best undertaken after appropriate chemotherapy and surgery to the limb. If lung metastases occur during or after treatment, then surgery is the most effective form of treatment and should be undertaken as soon as it is feasible. Modern techniques of operating on the lungs have greatly improved the ability of the surgeon to explore both lungs at the same operation, making it possible to remove metastases in both lungs.

RADIATION

In general radiation has nothing to offer in osteosarcoma and is used only to alleviate symptoms in terminal disease.

In Ewing's sarcoma, irradiation plays a major role in treatment of bones which cannot be surgically removed. For it to be effective, the doses of irradiation must be high and must include a margin of normal tissues. The undesirable effects of irradiation have been previously discussed. Nevertheless it may be the only effective modality for treatment of spinal canal and skull tumors.

In the past some oncology centers have used total lung irradiation for so called prevention of lung secondaries. The long term consequences of such treatment, as well as the improvements in chemotherapy and surgical techniques, have made this type of treatment outmoded.

There was also in the past a suggestion, that the brain and spinal canal should be irradiated due to the observation by one group of workers of involvement of these sites, in the same manner as in ALL (Chapter 10). Their findings have not been confirmed by other oncologists and this type of irradiation has been abandoned.

The irradiation approach that at present appears to be a reasonable compromise is the use of low dose irradiation after surgery. The advantage of this approach is that it reduces the long term undesirable consequences of irradiation.

RELAPSE

Lung metastases in osteosarcoma can be treated by lung surgery provided that the surgeon considers them to be operable. Chemotherapy is of value in those patients who have not previously received it. In patients who have developed metastases on chemotherapy, or after chemotherapy has been discontinued, further courses of chemotherapy have not been shown to be of benefit.

Lung metastasis in Ewing's sarcoma can be treated in a similar manner, but they can also be irradiated. For curative purposes, surgery, if feasible, holds out the best prospect.

Spread of either tumor to multiple bones is a dreaded type of relapse because in most instances it is incurable. Chemotherapy and irradiation can be very useful methods of pain control for variable periods of time. In Ewing's sarcoma total body irradiation with bone marrow transplantation has been used in a small number of patients with inconclusive results because of the difficulty in tumor control. Because osteosarcoma cells are insensitive to irradiation this type of approach is not useful in that tumor.

TERMINAL CARE

Most aspects of this subject have been discussed. Nowadays the most common cause of death in both tumors is multiple bone secondaries. These are very painful. Frequently the doses of morphine and its analogues required for pain control are so large that the patient is perpetually drowsy. An effective way of producing pain control without the use of large doses of morphine is direct infusion of the drug into the spinal canal. In children with bone pain, it is wise to adopt this approach sooner rather than later because it is more effective in controlling pain, and provides a better quality of life. There are some circumstances in the terminal care of these patients in which excisional surgery, or even amputation may be required for pain control, and this is a better option than uncontrollable bone pain.

CHAPTER 18

Muscle Tumors, Soft Tissue Sarcomas and Synovial Cell Sarcoma

The most common tumor in this group is that of the voluntary muscles of the body, and is known as rhabdomyosarcoma. This tumor has the microscopic appearance of primitive muscle cells and can arise in any part of the body in which there are muscle cells. Its embryonic nature, and the special genetic and possibly local environmental factors which give rise to these tumors, are highlighted by the peculiar sites of origin of so many of these tumors. While the great bulk of muscle fibres of the body is in the limbs, the back, neck and the posterior abdominal wall, the rhabdomyosarcomas more commonly originate from organs with a small muscle fibre component, such as the spermatic cord, the sinuses, orbits, middle ear, prostate, bladder and uterus.

A much less common tumor of muscles is one that arises from muscle fibres which are involuntary. These are known as smooth muscle fibres. These tumors are known as leiomyosarcomas and occur most often in the stomach.

The soft tissue sarcomas occur in areas of the body which contain supporting tissues and muscle fibres. These tumors often present in similar sites to rhabdomyosarcoma. The cells of these tumors lack the distinguishing features of rhabdomyosarcoma or the bone tumor known as Ewing's sarcoma. Because of this they are variously called soft tissue sarcomas, small round cell tumors, embryonal sarcomas or mesenchymal sarcomas. Their presentation, natural history and treatment are however very similar to rhabdomyosarcoma. The variant of soft tissue sarcomas known as synovial cell sarcoma is composed of cells which have a degree of differentiation which makes them distinguishable from the other soft tissue sarcomas. These tumors most often occur in the vicinity of joints or along tendon sheaths.

DIAGNOSIS

The clinical presentation depends largely on their site of origin. Most commonly attention is drawn to the tumor by its size and the pressure effects of the tumor on surrounding tissues, nerves and blood vessels. If the origin is in the eye socket (orbit), then there may be protrusion of the eye, swelling of tissues round the eye and squint. If the origin is in the sinuses, there will be swelling of a part of the face and possibly the inside of the mouth and paralysis of the nerves that supply the facial muscles (Bell's palsy). There may also be a persistent blood stained discharge from the nose. In tumors of the spermatic cord there may be unilateral enlargement of the testis, which may be mistaken for a hydrocoele or a hernia. Tumors of the bladder or prostate most often present in very young children with obstruction to urine flow. Sometimes it is noted that little fragments of tissue pass with the urine. Tumors of the vagina or uterus most often present with tumor tissue protruding from the vagina, or with obstruction to urine flow.

Tumors of the major muscle groups in the trunk or limbs are much less common than the ones discussed above, and usually present as enlarging but painless lumps. Sometimes these lumps are so big that they form ulcers. Occasionally the tumors are small and situated on the feet, but there is widespread tumor in the body. It is thought that the continuing massaging pressure on the tumor due to walking is responsible for the rapid spread of tumor cells from these relatively small tumors. There are many other unusual presentations of these tumors, all related to unusual sites of origin or the presence of metastatic disease.

The leiomyosarcomas usually present as an abdominal mass, possibly associated with partial bowel obstruction which causes vomiting. The soft tissue sarcomas, with the exception of synovial cell sarcoma, present in the same way as a rhabdomyosarcoma. The synovial cell sarcomas usually present as very painful swellings in the vicinity of joints or along tendons. A marked feature of these tumors in many patients is the extreme sensitivity, or even pain, on touching the skin over the tumor. This is known as hyperasthesia.

On the clinical suspicion that such a tumor is present, the extent of the tumor can be most accurately determined by CAT scans. Very often the true extent of the tumor is far greater than its superficial appearance. This is particularly true in tumors of the sinuses, pharynx and back of nose, and the middle ear. In these tumors it is essential to determine whether there has been spread into the central nervous system. This is determined by appropriate scans of the brain and the bones of the skull, as well as a spinal tap.

Once the true size and extent of local spread of the tumor has been established, its nature is determined by a biopsy. This is often undertaken only after staging procedures have been completed. The biopsy is examined under the microscope and the pathologist will name it according to its appearance as embryonal, alveolar or pleomorphic rhabdomyosarcoma. In the case of the other tumors it will be given one of the names previously discussed.

STAGING

Rhabdomyosarcoma has a tendency to metastasize to lymph nodes, lungs, bones and bone marrow. Whether it has spread to the lungs can be determined by a CAT scan of the lungs. Spread to bones can be detected by an isotope bone scan, and to the bone marrow by a bone marrow aspirate. Spread to lymph nodes is more difficult to ascertain, but it determines the type and extent of treatment. Part of the staging procedure may include a laparotomy with surgical exploration and biopsy, but not total removal, of lymph nodes. In practice laparotomy is only required in patients with paratesticular or lower limb muscle rhabdomyosarcomas.

The staging procedure for other soft tissue sarcomas and synovial cell sarcoma follows the same lines as for rhabdomyosarcoma. For leiomyosarcomas, extensive staging is usually not necessary because they metastasize less often.

PROGNOSTIC FACTORS

In rhabdomyosarcoma the most important prognostic factors are the site of origin of the tumor, the extent of spread, and the microscopic appearance of the tumor. These factors are closely inter-related. Thus tumors of the orbit, bladder, prostate, vagina and uterus have a very good chance of cure (approximately 80%), very seldom spread to other tissues, and are most often embryonal in microscopic appearance. Tumors of the sinuses and the back of the nose and throat frequently spread locally to infiltrate the bones of the skull, lymph nodes and even the brain. In about half the cases the tumors are alveolar or pleomorphic in microscopic appearance. Despite vigorous treatment the chances of cure are only about 30%. In tumors of the spermatic cord there is spread to lymph nodes in the abdomen in about half the patients, but it is rare to see spread beyond these glands. The microscopic appearance is mostly embryonal, and chance of cure is again very good (approximately 80%). Tumors of the major muscle groups have a high tendency to spread to lymph nodes, bones and lungs, are often alveolar or pleomorphic, and the cure rate is only about 40%. In patients presenting with widespread disease involving lungs and bones, the chances of cure are very poor irrespective of microscopic appearance or site of origin.

The prognosis of the soft tissue sarcomas is similar to rhabdomyosarcoma. These tumors often originate in tissues near major muscle groups, or in the chest cavity where there is difficulty in complete surgical excision. The cure rate is in the vicinity of 40%.

Synovial cell sarcomas are very aggressive tumors and the prognosis is only good if radical surgical procedures are used to excise the tumor. Minor surgery usually results in tumor recurrence and spread, leading eventually to death.

The leiomyosarcomas have a good prognosis, as in the majority of cases they have not spread to other tissues. However, if spread has occurred then the prognosis is poor.

TREATMENT

When the tumor is operable the major treatment modalities are surgery and chemotherapy. Surgery should be planned so as to excise the whole tumor with a margin of normal tissues. In practice, surgery is most often possible in the treatment of spermatic cord (paratesticular), and limb muscle rhabdomyosarcoma and intestinal leiomyosarcoma. Unfortunately, in the case of orbital rhabdomyosarcoma, surgery involves the removal of the eye.

The role of surgery in the rhabdomyosarcoma of prostate, bladder, uterus and vagina is much more controversial. If one were to undertake surgery at presentation it would require complete removal of these vital structures with disastrous life long consequences, such as an artificial bladder or the lack of reproductive organs. Because of this, surgery is delayed or used only for biopsy. The initial mode of treatment is to shrink the tumor with chemotherapy. After chemotherapy, assessment is made as to whether the tumor is operable without the removal of vital structures. If it is operable, surgery is undertaken and chemotherapy is continued. If the tumor is only operable by total removal of vital structures, surgery is not undertaken but instead irradiation is used for local tumor control. Irradiation to the pelvis also has major long term consequences related to arrest of growth and infertility, but it avoids the deformities of major surgery. Similarly, with tumors of the sinuses and back of nose and throat, surgery is so mutilating that its only role is that of biopsy. The only exception is rhabdomyosarcoma arising from the tonsil, in which case surgery can remove the bulk of the tumor without causing major deformities. In leiomyosarcomas surgery is the main form of treatment.

In synovial cell sarcomas, surgery offers the only chance of cure. In tumors which involve joints the only effective surgery is amputation or radical removal of the joint with surrounding bone, and bone and joint replacement. In other sites wide field excision of the tumor with a generous margin of surrounding tissues is essential.

Chemotherapy

In rhabdomyosarcoma this is used to reduce tumor bulk and prevent or treat disseminated disease. The mainstay of chemotherapy is a drug combination of vincristine, actinomycin–D and cytoxan which has the acronym of VAC. Adriamycin is sometimes added to this combination but its value is disputed. In cases of advanced tumors other drugs are often also incorporated into treatment programs. Ifosfamide, VP–16 and cis-platinum appear to be promising agents.

Special care has to be taken when the above treatment regimens are combined with irradiation because some of the drugs e.g. actinomycin–D and adriamycin potentiate the effects of irradiation on normal tissues, which may cause severe toxicity. In addition concomitant use of cytoxan or Ifosfamide with irradiation to the pelvis may cause bladder damage giving rise to hemorrhagic cystitis. To prevent these side effects, chemotherapy regimens are modified by withholding these drugs during, and for 4–6 weeks after irradiation.

In soft tissue sarcoma and synovial cell sarcoma, chemotherapy is an adjuvant to radical surgical excision. The chemotherapy regimens that appear to be most effective for these tumors are the same ones used for the treatment of Ewing's sarcoma. Chemotherapy is of doubtful value in leiomyosarcomas.

Irradiation

This plays a major role in local tumor control in rhabdomyosarcomas of the head and neck region, and those arising from pelvic structures. In head and neck rhabdomyosarcomas the irradiation may need to be given to the base of the skull and the brain if the tumor has infiltrated these structures. In almost all cases of head and neck irradiation there will be damage to the pituitary gland which controls hormone production. This will require hormone replacement therapy to assist with growth and pubertal development. In the case of rhabdomyosarcoma of the orbit, while surgery is successful in curing the patient, it does require removal of the eyeball. For this reason irradiation has replaced surgery and is equally successful in tumor control without the need to remove the eye. The long term consequences of irradiation of the orbit include retardation of growth of the orbit and the eye, cataracts and damage to the pituitary gland.

Irradiation of the pelvic structures is also preferable to surgical excision of these vital organs. The long term consequences of irradiation are retardation of growth of the pelvic bones, damage to the bones of the hip joint and sterility due to destruction of reproductive cells. Despite these undesirable sequelae, the fact that the pelvic structures remain intact, and normal sexual development and behavior can occur, makes irradiation the preferred treatment option.

In rhabdomyosarcomas of the spermatic cord and lower limbs a laparotomy is undertaken to see whether the tumor has spread to the lymph nodes of the pelvis or the abdomen. If such spread has occurred then irradiation of the lymph nodes in the pelvis and along the midline of the abdomen is used, as well as surgery and chemotherapy.

In the case of leiomyosarcoma, irradiation is seldom used unless there has been spread of tumor to lymph nodes in the vicinity of the tumor. In soft tissue sarcomas, irradiation is used in a similar manner to rhabdomyosarcoma. Irradiation is of no value in synovial cell sarcomas because the doses which are required to kill the tumor are so high that they also kill the underlying and surrounding normal tissues.

EMOTIONAL RESPONSES TO TREATMENT

Because of the sites of origin of these tumors, their treatment frequently results in some, often major, type of deformity of body image and function. Irradiation in the region of the face will result in facial asymmetry or even deformity. Irradiation of the pelvis will also result in some degree of deformity and sterility. Irradiation of a muscle group in the limb will interfere with the limbs growth. These long term consequences cannot be ignored and some form of rehabilitation is required to help children to overcome these handicaps. There is a variety of plastic surgery techniques and prostheses which can help such children to improve their appearance. Psychological support should also be used to channel the child's interest to areas in which their handicap will not prove a major disadvantage. Despite such measures it is wise to expect problems in adolescent and early adult years and to try and diminish these by the use of self help groups of young people with physical handicaps.

There are numerous national and international organisations of children with cancer in different age groups which can act as a source of support for young people with long term treatment sequelae. Most pediatric cancer centers have contacts with such groups.

CHAPTER 19

Brain Tumors

The brain is situated within the skull which protects it. The brain and the skull are lined by membranes which serve to anchor the soft substance of the brain to its appropriate sites in the skull. These membranes are known as the meninges. The skull has 2 major compartments. The anterior one, in which are situated the two major hemispheres of the brain known as the cerebral hemispheres and the posterior one called the posterior fossa, in which are situated the brain stem and the minor hemisphere known as the cerebellum. This is illustrated in Figure 8.

The posterior fossa communicates directly with the spinal canal through a hole in the skull known as the foramen magnum. Obstruction of the foramen magnum can interfere with the flow of the fluid which bathes the brain and is known as cerebrospinal fluid (CSF). CSF is actively produced by a group of cells which are closely associated with a bunch of blood vessels known as the choroid plexus. The choroid plexus secretes CSF into conduits in the brain known as ventricles from which the CSF exits to bathe the brain and pass down the spinal canal to bathe the spinal cord and its nerve roots.

Obstruction to the flow of CSF can occur as a result of blockage of the ventricles. This results in a build up of CSF pressure in the compartments in front of the obstruction, with distension of the ventricles, and compression of the nerve cells and supporting tissues of the brain adjacent to the ventricles. The medical term for this situation is hydrocephalus, and its symptoms are headache, vomiting and seizures. Severe degrees of hydrocephalus are life threatening because they push parts of the brain into the foramen magnum. The parts of the brain which impact in the foramen magnum have nerve cells which control heart beat and breathing, and their compression within the narrow and rigid foramen magnum may cause death.

In childhood some 60% of tumors arise in the posterior fossa. As a consequence of the anatomy, which has been previously described, these tumors often cause raised intracranial pressure, and tumor cells can readily pass through the foramen magnum to the spinal cord.

DIAGNOSIS

The most common presenting symptoms are those of raised-intra-cranial pressure. These are headache, vomiting and visual disturbance, and occasionally seizures. In addition, balance and limb movement coordination mechanisms are situated in the posterior fossa and may be damaged by the tumors. Thus, sudden onset of clumsiness, abnormal gait and frequent falls may be the first symptoms. In the case of tumors situated in the anterior cranial fossa, focal or generalized seizures may be the first presenting features. Other less common presentations include sudden onset of paralysis of a limb or one part of the body, and in rare instances, physical changes in the body associated with abnormalities of hormone production. These are usually due to tumors involving a part of the brain known as the pineal gland (see below), and most commonly present as premature onset of puberty.

The appearance of any of the above symptoms usually leads to a medical examination which reveals objective findings of impaired function of parts of the central nervous system, and the presence of raised intracranial pressure. These findings are used by the doctor to localize the likely site of the disease process. The presence, exact anatomical location, size and degree of hydrocephalus are shown by CAT or by magnetic resonance imaging (MRI) of the brain. These two relatively non-invasive modes of investigation have virtually totally superseded other far more invasive radiologic procedures, such as pneumoencephalograms and angiograms. However, for investigation of the possible spread of tumor to the spinal cord a myelogram may be required. This consists of an injection of an x-ray opaque dye into the spinal fluid, which may demonstrate the presence of masses within the spinal canal.

DISTRIBUTION AND TYPES OF BRAIN TUMORS

In childhood, 60% of brain tumors occur in the posterior fossa and arise from primitive undifferentiated cells called neuroectodermal cells. There are two main microscopic types, called medulloblastoma and ependymoma.

Much less common tumors of the posterior fossa are gliomas of the brain stem. Although, in strict cancer terms these tumors are not highly malignant, their situation in the brain stem makes them particularly dangerous and difficult to treat. The brain stem contains nerve cells which control vital functions such as breathing and the heart rate, and damage to these cells by growth of the tumor may cause death.

In the anterior cranial fossa, the majority of tumors arise from the supporting cells of the nervous tissue known as glial cells, and are called astrocytomas. They are graded according to degree of malignancy into high grade (malignant) and low grade (less malignant). Other less common types are the primitive neuroectodermal tumors (PNET) which are closely related to medulloblastomas, occasional pineal tumors which may affect hormone control, and rarely adult type tumors known as glioblastoma multiforme.

The anatomic site of the tumor, as established by CAT and MRI suggest the likely diagnosis, and the exact microscopic type is established at the time of surgery. In the case of brain stem tumors, surgery is rarely undertaken because of the proximity of vital nerve cells to the tumor, and the possibility of damaging them with surgery.

TREATMENT

The mainstay is surgery. Neurosurgery is a highly specialized discipline. For the most effective treatment of brain tumors, it is essential that the neurosurgeon has a special interest in brain tumors, and there are established mechanisms of coordinating surgical treatment with radiation therapy and chemotherapy. As in other childhood tumors, the best results are obtained by a plan of treatment formulated when the diagnosis is first established, and in which consultants in radiation therapy and chemotherapy are involved in planning the treatment together with the neurosurgeon.

The initial CAT and MRI investigations provide information on the degree of hydrocephalus and the resectability of the tumor. If the tumor is considered to be resectable, this will be the first form of treatment, and will also relieve hydrocephalus without the need to use mechanical shunts. If the tumor is considered to be inoperable because of its size or anatomic location, surgery will often still be required to obtain a biopsy sample of the tumor and to insert a mechanical shunt to relieve hydrocephalus. Inoperable tumors are then treated by other modalities, but "second look" surgery attempting complete tumor removal may follow the other forms of treatment.

Other Modalities of Treatment of Brain Tumors

In operable tumors such as low grade astrocytoma and pineal tumors, there is no need for other treatment modalities. In all the other tumors however, irradiation and, in the malignant primitive cell tumors, chemotherapy are also used.

Irradiation

This is a major form of adjuvant treatment in medulloblastomas, ependymomas, brain stem tumors and astrocytomas. The difficulties with irradiation arise from the long term effects on the developing brain and on growth. The younger the child, and particularly younger than 3 years, the more severe will be the side effects. These are:

1. Intellectual retardation produced by irradiation of the brain.
2. Reduced or absent production of hormones regulated by the brain.
3. Reduced growth of the spinal column resulting in a marked reduction in height.

For these reasons the dose of irradiation in young children may need to be drastically reduced or postponed. In very young infants (less than 12 months) brain irradiation will produce such profound intellectual retardation that it *should not be used.*

In children with medulloblastoma there is a high tendency for dissemination of the tumor to the spinal cord. In these children it is necessary to irradiate the cranium and the spine (craniospinal irradiation). As previously mentioned irradiation of the spine results in decreased growth of the spinal column, and the younger the child, the more profound will be the long term consequences on growth and appearance.

In older children irradiation of the cranium and spine is well tolerated and there are fewer long-term consequences, but it is still necessary to monitor hormone function, and some retardation of growth of the cranium and spinal column must be anticipated.

Brain stem tumors are treated with high doses of irradiation localized to the brain stem only. Irradiation has to be given with great skill, because swelling of the tumor as a result of cell damage by irradiation may result in pressure on surrounding nerve cells which maintain vital functions of the body.

In children with inoperable malignant brain tumors there is a tendency to undertake early irradiation. There is however, evidence from the treatment of other childhood tumors that irradiation is most effective in eradicating cancers, and therefore contributing to cure, when the tumor bulk is first reduced by surgery and chemotherapy. It seems reasonable to postulate that the same may apply to brain tumors. There is now a growing body of opinion which recommends, in such inoperable tumors, the use of aggressive chemotherapy before irradiation. It remains to be seen whether this type of approach will achieve a higher cure rate.

Chemotherapy

Brain tumors are the only malignancies of childhood where there is still controversy about the role of chemotherapy. There is incontrovertible evidence, that in recurrent malignant brain tumors such as medulloblastomas and ependymomas, chemotherapy can shrink the tumor with prolongation of life, but not cure. Similarly, in infants under the age of 1 year, chemotherapy and surgery have been used as the only modality of treatment, with some children surviving for at least 1 year with no evidence of tumor.

Such experience indicates that some medulloblastomas and ependymomas are sensitive to chemotherapy, but it does not prove that addition of chemotherapy to surgery and irradiation will improve the cure rate. Studies in the USA and Europe have addressed this problem by giving substantial numbers of children with malignant brain tumors relatively non-toxic chemotherapy after surgery and irradiation. After many years of observation, such studies demonstrate a 10–15% advantage for children given surgery, irradiation and chemotherapy, when compared to those treated with surgery and irradiation only. During the years that these studies were in progress much more aggressive chemotherapy combinations have been devised, and they have been used after surgery and before irradiation. It has not yet been established that the long term results of these new approaches will be better.

In most childhood cancer centers there is agreement that chemotherapy should be used in malignant brain tumors which include medulloblastomas, ependymomas, high grade astrocytomas, and primitive neuroectodermal tumor in the anterior cranial fossa. The simplest regimens are Vincristine and a fat soluble chemotherapeutic drug known as CCNU. There was also transient interest in the MOPP regimen described in the chapter on Hodgkin's disease. More recently however, more aggressive combinations are being used in which multiple agents are given in short succession over 24 hours such as the 8-in-one, and more recently 12-in-one regimens. The 8-in-one regimen uses methylprednisolone, vincristine, BCNU, procarbazine, hydroxyurea, cisplatinum, Ara–C and cytoxan. In other centers investigations are being undertaken on maximum tolerable doses of cis-platinum and the epipodophyllotoxin VP–16. Although these approaches to vigorous treatment of brain tumors are still experimental, it is hoped that they will increase the cure rates in these tumors.

Treatment of Non-malignant Tumors

These tumors are the low grade astrocytomas, the pineal tumors, and a tumor of the membranes lining the brain and the skull bones known as meningioma. In all of these tumors, surgery is the most effective treatment option. Irradiation is only used when surgery has been incomplete or impossible because of the anatomical location of the tumor.

PROGNOSIS

The five year survival rate for children with malignant tumors treated with surgery and irradiation is approximately 50%. In medulloblastoma, the 10 year survival rate decreases to approximately 30% and there is evidence that recurrences can occur even after 10 years. For the ependymomas and malignant astrocytomas, the 10 year survival rate is only slightly below 50%, indicating that these children are truly cured. In children with benign tumors, the survival rate ranges from virtually 100% for meningiomas, to some 70% in astrocytomas.

LONG TERM CONSEQUENCES OF TREATMENT

These have already been discussed in the section on irradiation. The consequences are those of scarring at the site of the tumor leading to epilepsy, and in some patients, residual damage of nerve function leading to some degree of palsy. Retardation of intellectual function, hormone production and growth are due to irradiation, and are most profound in youngest children. It is essential to anticipate these difficulties and to make appropriate plans for education and social activities for children who are thus disadvantaged.

CHAPTER 20

Retinoblastoma

This is a malignancy of the light receptor nerve cells of the eye known as retinoblasts. It is a prime example of a genetically determined tumor.

INHERITANCE

It has been shown that in every retinoblastoma so far studied there is a major or minor loss of genetic material on both chromosomes 13. This abnormality occurs only in the tumor cells. Furthermore, in a small group of patients with retinoblastoma and other congenital malformations including mental retardation there is absence of a segment of chromosome 13 in all cells of the body. These findings strongly support the "Knudson hypothesis", namely that in some tumors abnormality on one of a pair of chromosomes occurs during formation of the germ cells, and the abnormality on the second of the pair of chromosomes occurs by chance in the cells that form a tumor. In retinoblastoma these chromosome abnormalities involve chromosome 13.

In practice extensive family studies have shown the following:

1. With a family history of retinoblastoma and tumor in both eyes (bilateral) and less often one eye (unilateral) the chance of retinoblastoma in offspring of the parents or the affected child is 50%.
2. With bilateral tumors but no known family history of retinoblastoma there is a high probability that a germ cell abnormality of chromosome 13 has been passed on and the chance of retinoblastoma in the offspring is also 50%.

3. With no known family history of retinoblastoma and a unilateral tumor, the chance of passing on the retinoblastoma is about 10–15%. This lower figure is really a combination of two possibilities. One is that there was a germ cell abnormality on chromosome 13 passed on but not expressed in the family. If this were the case then the probability of "passing on" the condition would be 50%. The other possibility is that by chance both of the pair of chromosome 13 were affected by a mutation in the retinoblasts. In this case there is no tendency to inheritance of this tumor.

ANTENATAL DIAGNOSIS

Recently a number of research laboratories have synthesized or isolated genetic copies (gene probes) of the retinoblastoma gene on chromosome 13. These gene probes can be used to determine whether there are major or minor abnormalities on chromosome 13. If there is a family history of retinoblastoma and such abnormalities are present on chromosome 13 of the embryo then it can be assumed that there is a high risk of retinoblastoma.

DIAGNOSIS

The presence of an abnormality of the eye is often first noted by the parents because the pupil, instead of being black has a silver appearance and reflects light like a cat's eye. If there is a family history of retinoblastoma then the tumor will be diagnosed by a medical examination of the eye. Fortunately nowadays it is rare to see a child present with a bulging or even ulcerated eye as a result of tumor growth.

STAGING

Medical examination of the eye is undertaken by an eye specialist (ophthalmologist) and the appearance and extent of the tumor is noted and often photographed. The size of the tumor is graded on a scale of I–V with grade I being very small and grade V occupying virtually the whole eye.

Staging investigations are also required because the tumor can spread by direct backward extension along the optic nerve to the central nervous system, or by blood borne spread to the bones, bone marrow or lungs. Staging investigations consist of a bone scan, bone marrow aspirate, x-ray and CAT scan of the lungs and a spinal tap. In very large tumors which can only be treated by enucleation of the eye, staging is completed by careful microscopic examination of the optic nerve to see whether it had been invaded by retinoblastoma cells. Retinoblastomas that have invaded the optic nerve or the outside lining of the eyeball (sclera) are staged as grade VI.

TREATMENT

Surgery

The aim is to eradicate the tumors while preserving sight but this is only possible if the tumor has not already destroyed sight. In grade I–III tumors, local therapy to the tumor is given by the use of light coagulation, cryosurgery or irradiation. In grade IV tumors irradiation is the preferred initial mode of treatment if there is evidence that some sight has been preserved. In grade V tumors if vision is permanently destroyed the eye is enucleated but if there is evidence of some sight preservation then irradiation may be attempted. Grade VI tumors require enucleation.

In children presenting with bilateral retinoblastomas and the possibility of retention of some sight the treatment is either irradiation of both eyes or irradiation of the eye with the least tumor and enucleation of the worst affected eye. Unfortunately it is not uncommon for bilateral retinoblastomas to present with advanced tumor and no vision, in which case both eyes may need to be enucleated.

Irradiation

This is an important modality for local control of intermediate sized tumors. The irradiation fields are carefully planned to use lateral rather than front on radiation beams so as to minimize the dose of irradiation on the lens and thus decrease the size of the cataracts which always occur in later years. It is essential to prevent movements of the head during the irradiation, and in very young or uncooperative children short acting general anesthesia may be required to administer the irradiation. To assess control of the tumor the eyes are re-examined 4–6 weeks after irradiation and if there is any evidence of residual tumor, light coagulation is used to eradicate the tumor.

Irradiation is also used in grade VI tumors where the primary tumor has been treated by enucleation. Grade VI implies spread of tumor cells outside the confines of the eye and therefore surgery cannot be expected to have removed all tumor cells. Irradiation is given to the eye socket and the remnants of the optic nerve. While this is successful in eradicating tumor cells from the eye socket it has no effect on retinoblastoma cells that have invaded the central nervous system. In patients with this complication, intrathecal methotrexate and cranio-spinal irradiation may be used as for acute lymphocytic leukemia (Chapter 10).

Late Complications of Irradiation

Irradiation for small tumors is often complicated by development of cataracts but in general has few other serious side effects apart from retardation of growth of the eye and eye socket. These are usually easily concealed by appropriate eye glasses.

Where irradiation is used in large doses as in grace VI tumors there is substantial retardation of growth of the eye socket which may cause difficulty in retaining an artificial eye. In addition the irradiation may affect the pituitary gland which regulates body growth and sexual maturation. It is necessary to arrange consultation with endocrinologists for to prevent these side effects by appropriate replacement hormone treatment.

Chemotherapy

This has a role in treatment in patients with grade VI tumors or tumors disseminated to other organs. The two most effective agents have been cytoxan and adriamycin. They are usually used in combination, and good responses of lung and bone marrow disease have been documented. Central nervous system involvement has been treated with methotrexate alone, but the response is only transient.

A variety of agents has been used for local intra-ocular tumor control. None have demonstrated a better activity than irradiation or light coagulation.

REHABILITATION

With unilateral tumors, vision is preserved and is functionally normal. An artificial eye should be fitted into the empty socket as soon as possible after surgery and the artificial eye is changed as the child grows older and the eye sockets enlarge.

With bilateral tumors and absent or markedly impaired vision, provision must be made to provide educational and training facilities through the agencies that assist the blind. Adjustment to blindness in early childhood is remarkably efficient, and modern learning tools including Braille typewriters and computer boards as well as a growing variety of educational aids make it possible for such children to achieve their full educational potential.

PROGNOSIS

The long term cure rates for tumors which are limited to the eye are 80–100%. The outlook is worse in grade VI tumors with 60–80% cure rates. Disseminated disease to the central nervous system or bone has very low cure rates.

There is a markedly higher incidence of osteogenic sarcoma in patients with bilateral retinoblastomas. The quoted incidence rates vary from 4–59%. The lower figure is based on a survey of all genetic cases (bilateral and unilateral) undertaken in the UK with a followup of up to 18 years. The higher figure is from a survey in the USA and applies to bilateral retinoblastoma only, with a followup of up to 35 years. The possible relationship between abnormalities on chromosome 13 and osteogenic sarcoma has already been discussed (Chapter 17).

CHAPTER 21

Germ Cell Carcinomas and Hepatoblastomas

The germ cell carcinomas arise from cells called endodermal cells which line the yolk sac of the primitive embryo, and which are destined to become cells of the ovaries or testes. The primitive cells that do not take part in the formation of ovaries or testes mature into supporting tissues mostly at the bottom of the spinal column (called the sacro-coccygeal region), and occasionally in the thoracic spine region. Under rare circumstances, these germ cells undergo a malignant transformation giving rise to a tumor which contains various differentiated cells which form microscopic structures resembling those of normal organs (teratoma), as well as sheets of primitive embryonal cancer cells which can grow to a large size and spread throughout the body. Because of the origin of these malignancies they are also sometimes called yolk cell carcinomas, embryonal germ cell sarcomas, malignant teratomas, or endodermal sinus tumors.

The germ cell carcinoma cells retain the potential to secrete a number of products which are characteristic of the early period of embryonal life. These are a protein known as alpha fetoprotein (α–feto protein) and placental hormones such as the human chorionic gonadotropin (HCG). A variety of other minor fetal proteins and enzymes is also produced by these germ cell carcinomas. Their presence and levels can be measured in the blood stream, and provides an accurate assessment of the tumor bulk, which is not only useful in establishing the diagnosis, but also in following response to treatment.

The hepatoblastomas are primitive embryonal tumors of the liver. Like the germ cell carcinomas, these tumors secrete alpha-fetoprotein and can grow to a very large size in the liver and spread to other organs of the body such as the lung. In embryonal life the liver develops from cells in the midgut region which contain endodermal cells similar to those that migrate to the testes or ovary. When these embryonal cells become malignant, they also secrete alpha fetoprotein.

DIAGNOSIS

These are malignancies of early childhood often presenting before the age of 1–2 years, but also seen in teenage. Germ cell carcinomas of testes present as a painless firm swelling of the testicle which is readily visible. The same tumors of the ovary are much less obvious, and can grow to a very large size before they are noted as a lower abdominal swelling. Occasionally, attention is drawn to such an ovarian tumor because of a surgical complication, such as rupture of the tumor or twisting on its stalk. All too often these large tumors are widely disseminated by the time their presence is noted.

The sacro-coccygeal tumors may also present deceptively because of their location at the bottom of the spine. They may present with a swelling of the buttock which is incorrectly considered to be a bruise or an infection. At other times the tumor mass is so large that it presses on the rectum, and even the bladder, with retention of feces and/or urine. On other occasions the tumor can press on the nerves of the spinal cord giving rise to partial or complete paralysis of the legs, bladder and rectum. This may manifest as marked weakness of the legs, persistent dribbling of urine, and leakage of feces.

Children with hepatoblastoma usually present with a very large swelling of the upper abdomen. This causes them to have a protuberant abdomen and gives them a fat and healthy appearance. These tumors virtually never cause jaundice. Very occasionally there may be hemorrhage into the tumor, in which case the child has a tender large upper abdominal mass and is anemic.

When a germ cell carcinoma is suspected, its presence and extent is determined by CAT scans and ultrasound examinations of the pelvis and measurement of the levels of alpha-fetoprotein and HCG. In some cases a biopsy may be considered necessary, but most often the presence of a mass and raised alpha-fetoprotein is diagnostic of these tumors. Further investigations are to determine staging.

In hepatoblastomas an ultrasound of the liver and the level of alpha-fetoprotein will establish the diagnosis. Another investigation which points to hepatoblastoma is an exceedingly high platelet count on full blood examination. Sometimes it may be necessary to perform an arteriogram to outline the blood supply to the tumor and the liver so as to assess the operability of the tumor.

STAGING

Germ cell carcinomas and hepatoblastomas spread readily. Staging of the extent of dissemination requires CAT scans of the lungs, bone scan, and a CAT or ultrasound examination of abdominal lymph nodes. As previously mentioned the level of alpha-fetoprotein and/or HCG will serve as tumor marker and permit monitoring of the response to treatment.

PROGNOSIS

Germ cell carcinomas of testes, ovary or sacro-coccygeal region which are localized have an excellent prognosis, and are curable by chemotherapy plus surgery in more than 90% of cases. Similarly, hepatoblastomas which can be surgically resected and are localized to the liver can also be readily cured by surgery alone in approximately 80% of cases. In patients with disseminated disease, cure can be achieved in some 50–60% with vigorous chemotherapy and follow up surgery. The prognosis is worst in children with multiple bone secondaries or very many (more than 20) lung secondaries.

TREATMENT

Surgery

This is the most effective way of curing localized tumors if they can be completely resected with a margin of normal tissues. In practice this is most often possible in testicular germ cell carcinomas, hepatoblastomas and occasionally ovarian tumors. In the case of ovarian tumors it will be necessary to remove the whole ovary, but if the tumor is so large that removal of the fallopian tube and uterus is necessary, then surgery should be postponed until chemotherapy has been given. Chemotherapy is usually very effective and can reduce the extent of the surgery.

In sacro-coccygeal tumors it is seldom possible to excise the whole tumor at the time of presentation, and surgery is best postponed till after chemotherapy. When definitive surgery is undertaken it usually involves excision of the coccyx and possibly lower part of the sacrum. In children presenting with involvement of the nerves of the spinal cord which supply the lower limbs, rectum and bladder, resolution of the tumor can be better achieved by the use of chemotherapy than by attempts at partial removal of the tumor. In the rare case of a germ cell carcinoma of the thoracic region, surgical removal is often possible before chemotherapy is used. Surgery in hepatoblastomas involves partial excision of the liver. This is a major surgical undertaking requiring experienced surgeons working in optimum conditions, in which very low body temperatures (hypothermia) can be induced. The aim is complete excision of the tumor without damage to the remaining normal liver. Intensive care life support measures are required for some time after the operation.

In patients with disseminated disease to the lungs, surgery after adequate chemotherapy can be curative.

Chemotherapy

Dramatic advances in the treatment of these tumors have occurred by the introduction of combination chemotherapy consisting of vinblastine, cis-platinum and VP–16. This treatment regimen is often called the Eichorn regimen after the person who first demonstrated its extraordinary effectiveness in adults with a testicular tumor called seminoma.

In addition to the above drugs, these tumors are often also strikingly sensitive to adriamycin, cytoxan and actinomycin–D. For advanced tumors, combination chemotherapy regimens using the whole spectrum of effective agents are often utilized. While these regimens are toxic, and require very careful supervision of the undesirable effects on kidney function, hearing and the lining of the gut, they are remarkably well tolerated by even very young infants, and should be used when chemotherapy is indicated.

Chemotherapy plays the major role in the treatment of all unresectable and disseminated tumors. Its role in totally resectable tumors is more controversial. Some authorities prefer to give adjuvant chemotherapy in short courses to all such patients, claiming that this approach will prevent the appearance of metastatic disease. Others consider that monitoring with alpha-fetoprotein levels will permit early detection of metastases which can then be treated with chemotherapy. This approach will save many patients the unpleasant side effects of chemotherapy. A reasonable compromise is to adopt the wait and see approach in small tumors, and to use short courses of adjuvant chemotherapy in large tumors.

Irradiation

This plays only a minor role in control of these malignancies. It is occasionally required in sacro-coccygeal tumors which have failed to respond to chemotherapy. In patients with recurrent local disease or spread from an ovarian tumor to the peritoneum, irradiation after chemotherapy plays a major role in tumor control. It is also a useful in alleviating the pain of bone secondaries.

MONITORING RESPONSE TO TREATMENT

The close relationship between the number of malignant germ cells and the levels of alpha-fetoprotein and/or HCG, uniquely allow monitoring of response to treatment. The alpha-fetoprotein is only slowly eliminated from the body with a halving of its original amount over approximately 3–5 days. This means that when there is a very high starting level of alpha-fetoprotein, return to normal may only occur after many weeks. For instance, if the starting level was 20,000 microgram/liter and the normal level is less than 10 microgram/liter, then normal levels will be achieved only after 55 days. HCG has a shorter turnover time (less than one day), but in childhood germ cell carcinomas it is less often raised, and therefore it is a less useful for monitoring progress.

While the relatively slow elimination of alpha-fetoprotein is a disadvantage in monitoring resolution of the tumor, it is of advantage in monitoring recurrence of tumor. Production of alpha-fetoprotein by tumor cells leads to its rapid accumulation in the blood, and therefore it is a sensitive index of tumor recurrence.

In the case of hepatoblastomas, the alpha-fetoprotein levels may return to normal levels very slowly, or there may be a transient persistence of slightly elevated levels. This does not signify tumor persistence but reflects growth of normal liver cells which, prior to their maturation, produce low levels of alpha-fetoprotein.

EMOTIONAL RESPONSES

Involvement of reproductive organs such as the ovaries or testes by a malignancy is very naturally associated with concerns about future fertility and virility. These problems are compounded by the sequelae of treatment with irradiation and chemotherapy.

Removal of one testis or ovary will not decrease fertility or virility. If there are cosmetic concerns about the presence of only one testis, a prosthetic testis can be placed in the scrotum thereby giving the appearance that both testes are present. Chemotherapy has no effect on virility in either sex and no effect on fertility in females. Its effect on males is less certain, but it is unlikely to cause infertility in pre-pubertal males. Irradiation of testes or ovaries destroys fertility, and has a variable effect on virility. For this reason irradiation is an undesirable modality for the treatment of these tumors. If its use was unavoidable, then replacement hormone therapy will be required to induce puberty. Special counselling is required for such girls and boys to allow them to come to terms with their infertility. Such counselling should be delayed until replacement hormone therapy is started.

CHAPTER 22

The Histiocytic Disorders

These are loosely grouped disorders which appear to involve the scavenger cells of the body which are called macrophages. Some of these macrophages are fixed in certain tissues and have lost the ability to migrate, while others circulate in the blood, bone marrow and lymph. Three main diseases will be discussed, namely histiocytosis X, malignant histiocytosis and hemophagocytic reticulosis.

HISTIOCYTOSIS X

This condition is also known by the names of medical people who first described it as Letterer-Siwe disease, and Hand Schuller Christian disease. Other types of histiocytosis X are also known as eosinophilic granuloma because of their microscopic appearance. The term histiocytosis–X encompasses all of these conditions and is more accurate because it describes the predominant cell involved in the disease, and the subtitle X makes it apparent that there is much to be learned about it.

Histiocytosis X appears to be a disorder of fixed tissue macrophages present during early embryonic life in the external lining and supporting tissues of the embryo. These macrophages serve to protect the embryo from invasion by foreign cells and bacteria in the amniotic fluid. They have a characteristic appearance under the electron microscope and are known as the cells of Langerhans. It is these cells that are involved in the condition known as histiocytosis X.

Diagnosis

The disease characteristically presents in 3 different ways in 3 different age groups:

1. In children younger than 2 years, histiocytosis X involves skin causing a seborrhoeic widespread rash which characteristically involves the trunk and the scalp where it is often thought to be cradle cap (a severe form of dandruff). Medical examination shows enlarged lymph glands and frequently enlarged liver and spleen. These children are often very ill with fever, failure to gain weight, anemia and rapid breathing. The diagnosis is made by suspecting that the condition is present and by biopsy of the skin. Staging will be discussed later.
2. From the age of approximately 2–8 years the disease presents with painful lumps over bones, especially the skull. There may be also non-healing ulcers of the hard palate with erosions of gums and premature eruption of teeth. Occasionally there may be excessive thirst and marked urinary frequency, which is subsequently diagnosed as diabetes insipidus. Diagnosis is established by biopsy of involved tissues which are most readily accessible.
3. In children over the age of 8 years, the condition usually presents as a painful bone or bones in an otherwise healthy child, and the diagnosis is considered as being likely on the basis of a punched out hole in the bone on x-ray. Diagnosis is established by biopsy of the most readily accessible involved bone.

Staging

When a diagnosis of histiocytosis X is suspected, a number of investigations are required to determine the extent of the disease. The presence and number of bony lesions is determined by x-ray of the whole skeleton which in this condition is more accurate than a bone scan. Involvement of bone marrow is determined by bone marrow aspirate. Malfunction of liver is diagnosed by liver function studies, and involvement of the lungs by chest x-ray. If there is a suspicion of diabetes insipidus (failure of posterior pituitary function), then tests of the osmotic pressure of blood and urine will establish the diagnosis.

Prognosis

In general the prognosis is best in the older age groups. Disease of bones only very seldom progresses to more widespread disease, and virtually never causes death. Disease of bones with soft tissues may cause serious disabilities, but is seldom fatal. Disease in infants younger than 2 years is often fatal unless treated, and even with treatment 20% of patients die of the disease.

Treatment

Single bone lesions may be treated by surgical curettage or even injection of cortisone into the lesion. Multiple bone lesions, or lesions in vital bone areas such as the cervical spine or neck of femur cannot be adequately treated surgically. However, they do respond well to chemotherapy. A variety of regimens has been described in the medical literature. Vinblastine, prednisone, methotrexate and VP–16 have all been demonstrated to be effective in treatment of multiple bone lesions. Irradiation of multiple bones may be considered as an easy alternative and is certainly effective in controlling local disease, but there are significant long term undesirable consequences.

Disease involving bones and soft tissues requires chemotherapy for control of serious deformities. Occasionally surgery is also required to excise resistant residual lesions. The response to chemotherapy in soft tissue lesions is rapid, but bone lesions are slow to heal. Recurrences are common, and patience is required when relapses occur some months after stopping treatment. The most effective chemotherapy regimens have been those using vinblastine, prednisone, methotrexate and cytoxan or VP–16 and prednisone.

Disease in children younger than 2 years is the most resistant to treatment, and chemotherapy with one or other of the regimens described above is required for control of the disease. It is important to realize that the response to chemotherapy is slower than in the leukemias and lymphomas, and that there should not be too many early changes in the chemotherapy regimens.

Diabetes insipidus

During embryonic life a part of the outer lining of the embryo is folded inwards and becomes the posterior portion of the pituitary gland. This part of the outer lining contains tissue macrophages with bodies of Langerhans, and it is for this reason that the posterior pituitary gland may be involved in histiocytosis X.

The cells of the posterior pituitary produce a hormone called anti-diuretic hormone (ADH). This acts on the kidney to promote reabsorption of water. Damage to these cells in histiocytosis X causes a failure of production of ADH which results in excessive production of urine. The ensuing dehydration causes thirst. This condition is called diabetes insipidus and is totally different from the much more common diabetes mellitus (sugar diabetes). Neither chemotherapy or irradiation prevent or cure diabetes insipidus. The condition can be very effectively treated by a nasal spray of synthetic ADH.

Rehabilitation

Special measures are only required when hearing or the teeth have been severely affected. For children with hearing loss, hearing aids should be arranged. For children who lose primary or secondary dentition, dental bridges or even dentures may be required. Skin rashes heal without scarring and plastic surgery for residual skin disease is never required.

HEMOPHAGOCYTIC RETICULOSIS

This is a disease of higher malignancy than histiocytosis X and presents most often during infancy or in the first two years of life. In some patients it is an hereditary disorder inherited in a dominant manner. This means that the chance of subsequent siblings developing this condition is 1:2. There are, however, patients with this disorder without a family history, and where subsequent siblings are free of disease. Hemophagocytic reticulosis in these children usually appears in late infancy.

Diagnosis

The presenting features are high fever, pallor and skin rash. Medical examination shows marked enlargement of the spleen, and to a lesser extent the liver. Blood counts show low values of all elements. A bone marrow aspirate shows ingestion of white and red cells by macrophage cells, hence the name hemo(blood)phagocytic(ingestion). The condition may involve the central nervous system, in which case a spinal tap shows the presence of excessive numbers of macrophages. It is necessary to differentiate this condition from a similar presentation which may follow a nonspecific virus infection. The features of this post virus syndrome are that it occurs in older children with no family history of this condition, and the spleen is not usually markedly enlarged. The post virus syndrome resolves rapidly, although the patient may need a transfusion.

Prognosis

This is usually a fatal condition. While cures are reported, they are rare. Chemotherapy can prolong life, and in reported cures appears to have been instrumental.

Treatment

A variety of chemotherapy regimens has been used. Most of these have utilized multiple agents including cortisone, vinblastine and more recently VP–16. Neither irradiation or surgery have any role in treatment. Another new approach has been the use of bone marrow transplantation, but this is only possible if a tissue compatible sibling donor is available (Chapter 7).

MALIGNANT HISTIOCYTOSIS

This is an even rarer disorder of childhood, which is also highly malignant. Its features are a marked enlargement of lymph nodes, either in the chest cavity, neck or in the abdomen. There is often also a marked rash.

Diagnosis

Fever, rash and enlargement of lymph nodes are the main presenting features. There may be a reduction in all blood elements, but this is not a prominent feature. A bone marrow aspirate shows no specific features. The diagnosis is established by a lymph node biopsy. Malignant histiocytosis, like hemophagocytic reticulosis, can involve the central nervous system, and its presence there is diagnosed by a spinal tap.

Prognosis

Prognosis is variable, but cures following chemotherapy are documented.

Treatment

Vigorous chemotherapy with vinblastine, daunomycin, prednisone and more recently, VP–16, with the additional use of methotrexate for CNS disease, has resulted in cures. Treatment should be continued for at least 1 year. Neither surgery nor irradiation play any role in treatment.

Glossary

"Alternative medicine" - Unproven and untested methods of cancer treatment usually practised in an unscientific and uncontrolled manner.

ALL - Acute lymphocytic leukemia.

Allogeneic bone marrow transplant - Transplant from another individual.

AML - Acute myeloid leukemia, same as acute non-lymphocytic leukemia.

Angiogram - A radiologic technique that displays the blood vessels by introducing a radio-opaque dye into the vessels.

ANL - Acute non-lymphocytic leukemia, same as acute myeloid leukemia.

Ascites - Excessive amounts of free fluid in the abdominal cavity.

Autologous bone marrow transplant or rescue - Removal of the person's own bone marrow followed by its infusion.

Autopsy - Surgical and pathologic examination of the body and its organs after death. Also called Post-mortem.

Bone marrow aspirate - Suction of bone marrow, usually from hip bones, by means of a special needle and syringe.

Bone marrow transplant - Intravenous infusion of bone marrow cells.

Bone marrow trephine - Cutting and suction of a piece of bone marrow by the use of a special needle.

CAT scan - Computerized axial tomography.

Chromosomes - Structures in the nucleus of cells along which are arranged the genetic code i.e. the double helix DNA structure.

CSF - Cerebro-spinal fluid, the fluid surrounding the brain and spinal cord within the skull and spinal column.

Differentiation - Development of specialized functions by the cell.

DNA - Deoxyribose nucleic acid, the genetic code of inheritance. Each DNA molecule is made up of a 5 carbon sugar, a phosphate and one nitrogenous base.

Dysmorphy - Abnormal structure or symmetry of body.

Embryology - Study of the process whereby an infant is formed after conception.

Emesis - Vomiting.

Extramedullary relapse - Recurrence of leukemia in organs other than bone marrow.

Graft versus host disease (GVHD) - The disease resulting from transplanted immune cells in the donor bone marrow reacting against the tissues of the recipient of that bone marrow.

Haplotype - Cell surface antigen structure (HLA-A,B,C & D) determined by a chromosome inherited from the parents.

Hematuria - The presence of blood in the urine.

HLA - Human leukocyte antigens.

Hydrocephalus - Build up of CSF pressure in the brain causing compression and malfunction of normal brain.

Hyperdiploid chromosomes - More than the normal 46 chromosomes.

Laparotomy - A surgical procedure for inspection and biopsy of structure in the abdominal cavity.

Mantle - Type of radiation used in the treatment of Hodgkin's disease.

Medullary relapse - Recurrence of leukemia in the bone marrow.

Meningitis - Infection of the membranes lining the brain and spinal cord and separating it from bony structures.

Metastatic disease - Spread of cancer outside the organ of origin. Spread may occur by local extension, the lymphatic vessels or by the blood stream.

MLR - Mixed lymphocyte reaction, a method for testing donor compatibility in bone marrow transplantation.

MRI - Magnetic resonance imaging.

NHL - Non Hodgkin's lymphoma.

Oncologist - Medical person specializing in the treatment of cancer.

Oncology - The study of tumors.

Palliative treatment - A form of treatment aimed at relief of symptoms of the disease without attempting a cure.

Pleural effusion - Fluid in the chest cavity between the lungs and the chest wall.

Pneumoencephalogram - A radiologic technique in which the anatomy of the central nervous system is displayed by introducing air into the central nervous system.

Prognosis - The expected outcome of the disease process with or without treatment.

Relapse - Recurrence of the cancer either at its original site or at distant sites.

Remission - Disappearance of clinical and laboratory features of the cancer. Remission does not imply total eradication of cancer and is therefore not synonymous with cure.

Sanctuaries - Organ in which cancer cells are protected from exposure to chemotherapy given in standard dose by the intravenous, intramuscular or oral route.

Spinal tap (lumbar puncture) - Insertion of a fine needle into the spinal space and fluid surrounding the spinal cord.

Striae - Stretch marks.

Trachea - Wind pipe.

Unstable remission - A short lasting remission usually induced with extra treatment during the induction of leukemia.

Venepuncture - Insertion of needle into a vein.

Venous access - The ability to find veins suitable for venepuncture.

LIST OF MOST COMMONLY USED ANTI-CANCER AGENTS

General Class	*Usual Name*	*Usual mode of Administration*	*Malignancies in which most often used.*	*Major specific toxicity.*
Plant alkaloids	Vincristine or Oncovin	IV push	Leukemia, solid tumors all types	Damage to peripheral nerves, hair loss, constipation
	Vinblastine or Velbe	IV push	Histiocytosis X, Hodgkin's, Germ cell carcinomas	Bone marrow, rarely damage to peripheral nerves
	Vindesine	IV push	ALL	Rare damage to peripheral nerves
Epipodophyllotoxins	VP-16 or etoposide	IV infusion	Ewing's, Histiocytosis X, malignant histio-cytosis, AML	Bone marrow, mouth ulcers low blood pressure, allergic reactions
	VM-26 or Teniposide	IV infusion	Neuroblastoma, ALL and NHL	Bone marrow, mouth ulcers, low blood pressure, allergic reactions
Antibiotics	Actinomycin-D	IV push	Wilms' tumor, rhabdomyosarcoma, bone tumors	Mouth ulcers, rash, potentiation of radiation effect

	Daunomycin or daunorubicin	IV push	ALL, AML, NHL	Bone marrow, mouth ulcers, heart muscle damage (cardiomyopathy)
Anthracyclines	Adriamycin or	IV push or infusion	Neuroblastoma, NHL ALL, AML, bone tumors	As above
	Bleomycin	IV or IM	Bone tumors, Hodgkin's	Skin pigmentation, lung scarring
Alkylating Agents	Cytoxan or Endoxan or Cyclophosphamide	IV push or infusion	Bone tumors, soft tissue tumors, neuroblastoma, NHL, bone marrow transplantation	Bone marrow, bleeding from bladder (hemorrhagic cystitis) heart muscle damage (cardiomyopathy)
	Ifosfamide	IV push or infusion	Ewing's sarcoma, rhabdomyosarcoma, unfavorable histology Wilms' tumor	Hemorrhagic cystitis, rash, peripheral nerve damage
	Nitrogen mustard or Mustine	IV infusion	Hodgkin's disease	Bone marrow, irritation of veins, infertility
	Melphalan or L-PAM	IV infusion	Conditioning for bone marrow transplantation, neuroblastoma	Bone marrow, mouth ulcers, water retention, hair loss
	Busulfan or Myeleran	P.O.	Conditioning for bone marrow	Bone marrow, lung scarring, skin

			transplantation, chronic myeloid leukemia	pigmentation
	Cis-platinum	IV infusion	Bone tumors, brain tumors, germ cell carcinomas, liver tumors unfavor-able histology Wilms'	Damage to kidney function leading to salt and water imbalance, loss of hearing at high pitch
	Carboplatinum	IV infusion	As above	Bone marrow, less damage to kidneys on hearing
	m-AMSA	IV infusion	AML	Bone marrow, abnormal heart rhythm
Nitrosourears	B-CNU C-CNU	IV infusion P.O.	Brain tumors, Hodgkin's, brain tumors	Bone marrow, kidney function damage, liver damage
Anti-metabolites	Methotrexate	P.O.,IV,IM,IT	ALL, osteosarcoma NHL	Bone marrow, mouth and gut ulcers, liver damage, kidney function damage
	6-mercaptopurine or 6-MP	P.O.	ALL	Bone marrow, jaundice
	6-thioguanine or 6-T6	P.O.	AML	Bone marrow, jaundice
	Cytosine arabino-side or Ara-C	IV SC	AML, NHL, ALL	Mouth ulcers, conjunct-ivitis, skin rash, damage

				to coordination of limb movements.
	5-fluorouracil or 5FU	IV push	Liver tumors, germ cell carcinomas	Mouth ulcers
	5-hydroxyurea 5-HU	P.O.	CML	NIL
Enzymes	Asparaginase	IM, S.C., IV	ALL, NHL	Diabetes, pancreatitis, disturbances of the blood clotting mechanism leading to excessive bleeding or to thrombosis, allergic reactions
Hormones	Prednisone	P.O. or IV	ALL, NHL Hodgkin's	Weight gain, diabetes, reduced response to infections, mood changes, muscle and bone wasting, peptic ulcers.

Index